S0-BMU-153

CRISES OF FAMILY DISORGANIZATION
Programs to Soften their Impact on Children

SOCIAL PROBLEMS SERIES
Sheldon R. Roen, Ph.D., Editor

Program Evaluation in the Health Fields
Edited by Herbert C. Schulberg, Ph.D., Alan Sheldon, M.D., and Frank Baker, Ph.D.

Psychiatric Disorder and the Urban Environment: Report of the Cornell Social Science Seminar
Edited by Berton H. Kaplan, Ph.D. in collaboration with Alexander H. Leighton, M.D., Jane Murphy, Ph.D., and Nicholas Freydberg, Ph.D.

Research, Planning, and Action for the Elderly: The Power and Potential of Social Science
Edited by Donald Kent, Ph.D., Robert Kastenbaum, Ph.D., and Silvia Sherwood, Ph.D.

Crises of Family Disorganization: Programs to Soften Their Impact on Children
Edited by Eleanor Pavenstedt, M.D. and Viola W. Bernard, M.D.

Retirement
Frances M. Carp, Ph.D.

Identifying Suicide Potential
Edited by Dorothy B. Anderson and Leonara J. McClean

Two, Four, Six, Eight, When You Gonna Integrate?
Frank A. Petroni, Ph.D., and Ernest A. Hirsch, Ph.D. with C. Lillian Petroni

CRISES OF FAMILY DISORGANIZATION
Programs to Soften their Impact on Children

Eleanor Pavenstedt, M.D. and
Viola W. Bernard, M.D., Editors

Papers delivered to the
New York State Fifth Biennial Divisional Meeting
of the American Psychiatric Association,
November 18, 1967

BEHAVIORAL PUBLICATIONS New York

Library of Congress Catalog Card Number 74-140052
Standard Book Number 87705-019-8

BEHAVIORAL PUBLICATIONS, 2852 Broadway—Morningside Heights, New York, New York 10025

Printed in the United States of America

Contents

Contributing Authors

Courtenay L. Bennett, M.D., *Assistant Director, Hudson River State Hospital; Commissioner of Mental Health, Dutchess County**

Viola W. Bernard, M.D., *Clinical Professor of Psychiatry, College of Physicians and Surgeons; Director, Division of Community and Social Psychiatry, Columbia University.*

Elizabeth Elmer, M.S.S., *Director of Infant Accident Study; Research Instructor, Department of Pediatrics, University of Pittsburgh School of Medicine.*

Ethel L. Ginsburg, A.C.S.W., *Staff Consultant, Citizens Committee on Children of New York, Inc.*

Roberta Hunt, M.S.W., *Consultant on Implementation, Community Council of Greater New York.*

Lillian C. Lampkin, M.S.W., *Assistant Professor, Hunter College School of Social Work; formerly Executive Director, New York City Youth Board.*

Charles A. Malone, M.D., *Training Director, Philadelphia Child Guidance Clinic, Associate Professor of Clinical Child Psychiatry, University of Pennsylvania Medical School.*

Eleanor Pavenstedt, M.D., Staff, Child Psychiatry, and Director Infants and Toddler Program, Tufts-Columbia Point Health Center; Lecturer, Tufts Medical School; Clinical Professor of Psychiatry, Boston University School of Medicine; Lecturer, Wheelock College.

* The professional positions of the contributors are listed as of 1968

Foreword

At the New York State Fifth Biennial Divisional Meeting of the American Psychiatric Association, held in New York City in November, 1967, the overall title for the program was: "Social Crisis and the Psychiatrist." The Program Committee Chairman was Louis Linn, M.D.

As part of the program, there were four workshops, held simultaneously. Section III dealt with "Problems of Childhood and Youth." In this Section, Workshop B was moderated by Dr. Viola W. Bernard; the Reporter for this Workshop was Dr. Alan M. Levy.

It is the papers in this workshop that are being published in this volume, under three subheadings: "Parents with Mental Illness," "Parents under Unmanageable Stress," and "Programs to Assist Parents." Dr. Eleanor Pavenstedt has written an introduction for each section.

The contributors are professional persons of national repute, who have devoted a great deal of their professional lives to the problems under discussion. The collection in one volume of the ideas of these professionals from the disciplines of psychiatry and social work is a major contribution. It is to be hoped that the material in this book will stimulate other workers throughout the country to initiate or expand programs similar to those described here.

The importance of this group of papers has been officially recognized by the Officers of the New York State Division of the American Psychiatric Association, and they have issued an official imprimatur for this purpose.

Frank J. Curran, M.D. November, 1967

Chairman, Section III, Childhood and Youth, Fifth Biennial Divisional Meeting, New York State District Branches, American Psychiatric Association.
Attending Psychiatrist, St. Luke's Hospital, New York. Former President, New York County District Branch, American Psychiatric Association.

Section 1

Parents with Mental Illness

Introduction

Dr. Viola W. Bernard and Mrs. Ethel L. Ginsburg express once again their concern over the absence of integration between the hospital staff caring for the psychotic parent and community agencies, which most of the time are not alerted to the plight of the patients' families or of the discharged patient. A follow-up study of the fifty examples gathered in 1962, referred to by both authors, would without any doubt bring to light sufficient evidence of tragic consequences of community neglect to add to the force of these voices crying in the wilderness.

That the Citizens' Committee for Children of New York has had an impact on the Mental Health Services of Dutchess County is clearly demonstrated by the third chapter of this section. The ingenious stroke of appointing the author, Dr. Courtenay L. Bennett, to both the county Inpatient and Day Care services (connected with but decentralized from the State Hospital) and to the Mental Health Services for the county has certainly contributed to the successful collaboration of all the services. This is amply exemplified by the family care reports included. Mental Health Centers will probably do well to concentrate overall responsibility and authority in the hands of one energetic, clear-headed, and devoted professional. Such a person will soon enough recognize his limitations in such fields as child psychiatry, psychosomatic medicine, court psychiatry, and psychiatry of the aging, and will obtain specialized personnel wherever possible.

Dr. Bennett's assurance that children already adversely affected receive family therapy leads us to be less concerned about the fact that only the infant's malnutrition is mentioned in the first example. Emotional sustenance, the opportunity to relate to a responsive mothering adult, is now known to be an essential ingredient for normal development during these months. In the second case, too, a psychiatric evaluation of the three children, aged 4, 8, and 12, together with attention to their developmental level and emotional impact on them of the mother's illness, suicide attempt, and separation, might have disclosed a need for therapeutic or preventive measures or both. This is not a criticism of what goes on in Dutchess County but merely a reminder of where we must set our sights.

Chapter I

Young Children of Mentally Ill Parents: Part I

Viola W. Bernard, M.D.

As we have come to view the family as a social system, we have also recognized that overt mental illness on the part of any one member of a family is not only a crisis of psychic disorganization for the index patient, but also a psychosocial crisis for all members of the family.

When the patient is a parent, his or her illness is highly likely to precipitate some measure of crisis for the children—especially for the young children in the family. The theme of this entire meeting, "Social Crisis and the Psychiatrist," and of this particular workshop, "Crisis of Family Disorganization," provides an opportunity to discuss some of the stresses for children resulting from parental mental illness, as well as ways of reducing the risk of its having damaging effects on them—effects that may range from a less obvious adverse impact on their emotional development to gross injury and neglect.

Recent developments in community psychiatry have offered the promise of closer integration, conceptually and at the service level, of measures directed toward the social and clinical aspects of mental illness. As yet, however, we are still far from achieving, or even recognizing, the necessity for adequate communication and coordination between the many professional sectors responsible for one or another of the services that are needed by the patient's family as a whole. Thus, psychiatrists in mental hospitals focus mainly on the parent-inpatient as they see him—that is to say, removed from his or her accustomed social contexts—somewhat in contrast to those community-based psychiatrists, for example, who function in day hospitals and in outpatient clinics. Meanwhile, child care personnel and child psychiatrists deal, in separate settings, with widely varying effects on the children of parental mental illness, as well as with the many kinds of crises such illness may entail for them—crises of separation and disruption, for example, when a mother is hospitalized, or of traumatic day-to-day exposure at home to her symptomatology.

In view of the ongoing interrelationships between parents and children within a family, optimal service would seem to call for corresponding interrelationships between the various professionals and agencies that are involved in dealing with parent-patients and their children; or, to put it more urgently, improved mechanisms of coordination and collaboration do seem essential in order to prevent or mitigate damage to large numbers of children—a problem that seems to some of us to have reached crisis proportions.

Before going any further, let me tell you about some of the background activities of the Citizens' Committee for Children of New York, Inc. with regard to this issue. The Committee is a voluntary organization of lay and professional persons concerned with the various interrelated aspects of children's services: health, mental health, protective services, education, childrens' rights, and so on. Both Mrs. Ginsburg, whose discussion will follow mine, and I have long been associated with this Committee. She is Staff Consultant, and I have been a member of its Mental Health Section.

In 1961-1962, the Committee, through a subcommittee of its Mental Health Section,* took the initiative of convening two meetings of eighty representatives from some thirty state and local health, mental health, and welfare services, voluntary and public—representatives who had policy-making and ad-

* Dr. Peter B. Neubauer and I were at that time co-chairmen of the Mental Health Section, and the other members of the subcommittee, who contributed greatly to the ideas on this subject then and since, were Drs. Grace Baker, Lauretta Bender, Abraham Lurie, Exie Welsch.

ministrative responsibility for the ambulatory and inpatient psychiatric treatment of adults and children, as well as for child welfare services.

The purpose of these meetings was to sound the alert on a problem that was in fact the common concern of all those who had come together, yet had not always been recognized as such, because so many of us were functioning in our own settings, without sufficient awareness of how what happened in one was able to help or hinder what could be accomplished in the other. Thus, by bringing into focus the risks and needs of children in relation to their parent's hospitalization, we hoped to help effect improvement in joint planning and in the treatment of both. In addition, the meetings sought, as a major aspect of their deliberations, to identify those potential hazards for young children that might be on the increase, as a side effect of profoundly important advances in chemotherapy and in community psychiatry, whereby increasing numbers of psychiatrically sick or vulnerable parent-patients were remaining in the community. We welcomed the many ingredients of the community psychiatry "movement," as it is sometimes called, that were making possible earlier discharge for many psychotic parents and reducing the social breakdown syndrome that often resulted from prolonged custodial hospitalizations. We recognized, too, the value of providing, within the community itself, a wider range of therapeutic alternatives to hospitalization, with a resultant more selective use of hospitalization.

What we sought to stress was that, if one looks at the program holistically, there may be a dangerous by-product, in terms of risks to young children from living at home in the care of psychotic parents in varying states of disturbance—some being maintained on drugs or other aftercare measures, some with no follow-up care at all, but all, to some extent, psychiatrically "vulnerable." We had no wish to set the clock back, to undo our own professional progress, which enabled the reduction of needless or over-prolonged hospitalization. We did feel, however, that as more psychotic parents, especially mothers, came to remain in the community, there would be a proportionate increase of various hazards resulting from close continuous contact as compared with those that were due to separations because of hospitalization. We believed that such a shift in the kinds of crises that children are actually facing should be recognized and measures should be taken to offset it by concerted efforts on the part of the professional and lay community. The basic idea of the meetings was to explore ways and means of supporting family resources so as to prevent, or at least minimize, psychologically harmful interactions when sick parents and their children remain at home together.

The Citizens' Committee undertook an initial canvass of the problem; surveyed the existing literature* (1) which was rather sparse; and tried to perform the social actions of identifying the problem, breaking down some of the communication barriers between those responsible for interconnected forms of care, and stimulating further study and service development. At the request of those who attended the first of the two meetings, we formulated a report in 1962 (2) that tried to put together some of the thinking about this problem. In that report, we indicated the magnitude of the problem and offered documentation as to its urgency, by way of fifty vignettes of children who were known to the various agencies whose representatives attended the original meeting. These illustrative case vignettes were truly horrifying, in terms of how young children were suffering in ways that were associated with the chronic or acute mental illness of a parent (particularly when the parent was the mother)—not only as the result of separation due to parental hospitalization and its attendant crises, but also from continued or intermittent contact with sick parents at home.

We strove to emphasize in that report, and I want to stress again on this occasion, five years later, that by no means should we imply, nor does the evidence support, the existence of a simple one-to-one relationship—that is, that the psychiatric

---

* A "Digest of Recent Literature on Children of Mentally Ill Parents" was prepared by Miss Rose Goldman, a member of the Mental Health Section of the Committee, in 1962.

illness of parents *necessarily* impairs their parental functioning, with inevitable damage, therefore, to their children's mental health. Such a conclusion is not borne out by the facts. Some parents are afflicted, however, in ways that do impair their parental competence and which seriously interfere with meeting their children's needs for healthy development and emotional well-being.

In other instances, psychotic mothers appear to be able to maintain affectionate relationships with their young children and to take good care of them. The point is that a great many variables—some pertaining to the child, some to the psychotic parent, to other family members, and to situational factors—determine whether or not there is a detrimental relationship between the psychoses of parents and the development and adjustment of the young children they rear in the course of intimate daily contact. Therefore, in view of the vulnerability of these young children and the evidence that they may be at special risk of suffering gross to subtle forms of psychic harm, it seems urgent that there be a suitable psychosocial evaluation in each case of parental illness from the standpoint of possible damage to children's mental health, and further, that significant weight be given such evaluation in the treatment plan for each parent-patient. Moreover, as with aftercare, periodic family-focused appraisals are called for, so that changing indications for therapeutic interventions or for other forms of assistance may be recognized and implemented.

It should be clear that, in recommending differential individual assessments on which to base differential modes of safe-guarding these children, we would regard it as totally unjustified to approach the problem with such policies as a regression to the over-hospitalizing of adults, or by the routine removal from the home of children whose mothers are, or have been, psychiatrically ill. Children should certainly not be placed in foster homes—of these there already exists a serious shortage in relation to true need—unless such placement has been clearly established as the plan of choice. The damage of separation from the mother, other family members, and the home surroundings must be weighed, in each particular instance, against the damage from disturbances in the mother-child relationship that have been induced as the result of the former's illness.

We also know that there are many vulnerable parents among those who are discharged from mental hospitals or who stay in the community, who may be enabled to give adequate nurturance to their young children in spite of their possessing at best a marginal parental competence—if this is sufficiently *supplemented* by timely and pertinent social, economic, and psychological supports. Thus, it can make a critical difference in their capacity for mothering if relief from child care is provided, for at least some hours of the day, by a day care center; or if there are relatives to lend a hand, or if the husband—provided there is a husband—can carry enough of the load; or if there are older children in the family who are able to help; or if homemaker service is provided; or if there is appropriate counseling or economic assistance.

Sometimes a baby or toddler feels the main impact of a parent's mental disorder indirectly through the stressful effects it has on the other family members—effects that impair how they care for and relate to him. It follows, therefore, that stress-relieving help to his non-psychotic parent and siblings may be, for such a little child, a most effective, even though indirect, form of emotional protection.

Of course it is time-consuming, and it calls for a high degree of knowledge and skill, to carry out the sort of family evaluations we have urged, and to differentiate diagnostically the young children and their needs. In fact, one of the more serious deficiencies in the training and consequently in the professional abilities of many, if not most of us, in child psychiatry and in its related fields, has to do with the diagnosis and treatment of developmental problems and deviancies among infants and pre-school children. Consequently, planning for their care is often too manipulative, as though they were inanimate pawns rather than individually differing sensate beings. Of course, this professional deficiency needs to be corrected for many other reasons besides the purpose on which we are focusing here; yet this purpose does lend added urgency to developing and training workers in this field in methodologies that permit more accurate assessment with this age group than the rather crude methods that are now commonly used.

We are under no illusion about the formidable difficulties, of many kinds, that would have to be overcome in order to actually bring into being—in terms of both quality and quantity—the sort of multi-service programing that we have been advocating in these remarks. Are the needs that we have indicated borne out by research findings? By way of what kind of organizational and administrative patterns can the necessary coordination and communication be brought about among the great variety of agencies and categories of staff involved? Can problems of manpower training and supply, as well as of funding, be overcome? Is there evidence to indicate the effectiveness of such approaches? And, of crucial importance, how would the families for whom these services are intended feel about making use of them.

As yet, only partial answers can be given—some, to be sure, more fully than others—and in this very brief paper, I shall not even try to marshal the data already available that do bear on these questions. Instead, I shall touch on just a few of them, in keeping with the purpose of today's panel, which, as I understand it, is primarily to *identify types of crises that should be of concern to psychiatrists* and to galvanize our efforts to help resolve these crises. We hope, therefore, that this discussion will be able to stimulate the further research, demonstration projects, program evaluation, and innovations in the delivery of coordinated services to young children and their parents that seem to us to be warranted by research and experience thus far, and which will surely be needed if we wish to arrive at more complete answers to the questions that have been raised here. *

* It is encouraging to note the progress along these lines that has occurred since the presentation of this paper. Thus, at a single meeting of the American Psychiatric Association in 1968, preliminary reports of *four significant*

In 1962, Ekdahl *et al.* (3) made a pioneering contribution by drawing attention to the crises that the hospitalization of parents entailed for their children and families. As compared with the children of parents who had been hospitalized for tuberculosis, the youngsters of psychiatrically hospitalized parents were found to suffer much more neglect and abuse; they were also often felt by psychotic parents to be involved in the latter's delusional symptoms, and they had undergone a great deal more disruption in living arrangements and patterns of care. The crises for the children were greater when it was the mother, rather than the father, who was hospitalized, while children in one-parent families suffered the greatest disruption and seemed the most in need of community resources. The authors concluded that "The inference to be drawn from this study is that the combined resources of mental hospitals and

---

investigations were presented, each exploring in more sophisticated and thorough ways than most of the studies to date, highly relevant aspects of needed knowledge in this area. Of these four contributions, the following two seem especially germane:

Gallant, Grunebaum, and Weiss presented a critical review of the literature dealing with psychosis in parents, particularly in mothers, in relation to developmental deviations in children. These authors have emphasized the research value of determining how *specific aspects of the mother's illness and personality* can be related to specific deviations in the child, and the importance of such study design to the problem of evaluating preventive intervention programs. These authors, along with two more colleagues, have intensified and expanded their work, which is to be reported in a book, *Mentally Ill Mothers and Their Children,* to be published in 1971 by University of Chicago Press.

At the same meeting, Anthony outlined a five-year study of the children of psychotic parents with control cases drawn from families in which parents have needed hospitalization for chronic physical illness. As Anthony states, "Careful clinical evaluation can bring to light a spectrum of disturbances manifested by children associated with high risk psychotic heredities and high risk psychotic environments." Anthony points out sources of error in the absence of careful and thorough clinical appraisal, as accounting for the frequency of negative findings of children's mental health on the basis of school or agency assessments. As he puts it, "The farther the research distance between investigator and child, the more likely is the latter to be rated high on adjustment."

community health and welfare services at present fail, for the most part, to deliver significant help to children of hospitalized parents." This study did not focus primarily on the very young children in these families, nor did it concern itself mainly with those children whose psychotic parents are maintained for the most part in the community, as we are doing today. It did recognize, however, that the patterns of mental hospitalization were changing rapidly, and that there was a consequent need for new ways of combining and expanding hospital and community responsibility toward the children of mentally ill parents.

Sobel (4) has conducted one of the few studies so far of infants of psychotic parents. His sample was admittedly small. Of the eight infants whose early development he observed, each had two schizophrenic parents; four of these babies were placed in foster homes and four were reared by their schizophrenic parents. Three of the latter four developed clear-cut signs of depression and irritability, whereas none of the four who were reared in foster homes showed any signs of developmental problems, as judged by observations made in monthly home visits. According to Sobel, "Our data suggest that the parental behavior of their schizophrenic mothers was at least partially responsible for the early emotional maldevelopment observed in these three infants."

A 1966 Maudsley monograph, *Children of Sick Parents, an Environmental and Psychiatric Study* by Rutter (5) is extremely germane to our need to learn more about the effects on children of overt parental mental disorder, especially in view of recent trends toward the community care of psychiatric patients, and the consequent increase of interactions between psychotic parents and their children at home. The book includes a discerning review of the literature; it contrasts, for example, the conclusions of those authors who assume it to be better for children that their psychotic parents be out of the home and in hospital, with others who take the opposite view, seeking to protect children against "family break-up" and long separations from their mothers. As a critical factor in this regard, Rutter points out the extent to which maternal separation effects are now known to depend on the quality of substitute care.

He studied 922 children who had attended the Maudsley Psychiatric Clinic, in terms of the extent and nature of mental illness among their parents. He also investigated the extent of chronic and recurrent physical illness among the parents of these "disturbed" children, using as a control group children who had attended dental and pediatric outpatient clinics. His study seems to be particularly valuable because of the range of variables it deals with, which makes it possible to ask more differentiated questions of the data. Among the findings that are of the greatest relevance to our topic is an association between parental mental illness and psychiatric disorder in the children. He concluded that the genetically determined heightened susceptibility to psychiatric disorder, on the part of children of mentally ill parents, is unlikely to be the major factor in the association; rather the disorder in the child must be viewed as *one consequence of the impact of parental illness* on the family.

Rutter also concluded that not all parent illnesses lead to deviant development in the children; further, when there are harmful consequences, not all children are affected equally, children differing in their susceptibilities in this regard. One important finding was that the seriousness of the parent's psychiatric disorder seemed less significant than whether or not the child was involved in the symptoms of the parental illness. ". . . Delusions per se do not matter particularly but if the delusions directly involve the child and affect the parental care, it seems that the child is more likely to develop a psychiatric disorder." Rutter's data also indicate that, with a number of parental emotional illnesses, it is the youngest children who are at the highest risk of developing disturbances.

Sussex *et al.* (6) studied the adjustment of sixteen children, aged six to ten, who lived at home with psychotic mothers. Although the authors recognized the need for a larger sample, a longer period of observation, and better criteria for assessing the quality of parental functioning, their finding was that these latency-aged children showed minimal adverse effects; they did, however, stress that these psychotic mothers were receiving outpatient treatment. Even so, the younger the child, the greater was the adverse influence upon him; on the other hand, the risk of adverse effects was decreased if family resources were available to assist the psychotic mother in continuing to function or to substitute for her when illness impaired her mothering role.

Higgins (7) studied two groups of twenty-five children, each born to schizophrenic mothers; the children in one group were reared by their mothers, those in the other were reared from an early age "by agents without a history of psychiatric illness." He reports that the results failed to support his initial hypothesis—namely, that the children who had been reared by their own mothers would display greater maladjustment than would those children who had been reared by others, when both were evaluated by various measures at fifteen years of age. However, without knowing more—for instance, about the substitute mothers and the quality of care experienced by the reared-apart group; the mother-infant interactions of this group with their own schizophrenic mothers before separation, which occurred at the mean age of one year seven months, and some differentiation within the global category of schizophrenia—it would seem unwarranted to interpret these findings to mean that young children of mentally ill parents are not at special risk, or to relax efforts to provide better protection for them in connection with treatment planning for the sick parent and available supports for the family as a whole.

It may be worthwhile to review, for use in future planning of service programs, a few of the reported attempts to mitigate the crises of parental mental illness for children in families. In 1966, Rice and Krakow (8) * reported on a demonstration

---

* Since then, not only has another study in this series been reported (Ekdahl, M. C. "Limitations of Emergency Services for Mentally and Emotionally Disturbed Mothers." *Am. J. Pub. Health,* **60,** July, 1970), but the valuable corpus of work by these investigators will be issued in book form—*Children of Mentally Ill Parents,* E. P. Rice et al.—by Behavioral Publications about the same time that they also publish this volume on family crises.

study, undertaken on the basis of an earlier study report, of which Miss Rice was a co-author. In the demonstration, families of parent-patients from one town that was served by the nearby State hospital were referred, as soon after admission as possible, to the project's community coordinator. Through interagency cooperation, these forty demonstration families were able to receive a variety of immediate, continuous, and coordinated service, while the families of fifty-nine parent-patients from other towns served by the same hospital were not referred to the community coordinator for assignment to a key agency, but instead received only such services as were regularly available to them on their own request.

Findings were reported in relation to child care, the mental hospital, and the community. The return of the ill parent to the home often created new problems in the care of children, since the mothers involved might not be ready to assume the responsibilities of caring for their children; it was the younger children who experienced the greatest amount of separation, many of them being shifted from one caretaker to another, in a relatively short period of time. Homemaker services proved to be of value in supporting both relatives and those mothers who had been discharged from the hospital. Although families had tended not to request agency services at the time of the parent's hospitalization, most of them did welcome the services provided by those agencies that reached out to them. The authors found that new methods of providing prompt intervention, interagency collaboration, and hospital community co-operation were tested and found effective, but they concluded, nevertheless, that "Additional methods and skills appear to be required to achieve adequate protection of children with mentally ill parents either at home or in the hospital."

Coleman (9) in 1967 reported on another, more extensive five-year care project undertaken jointly by a State mental hospital and four community-based agencies—an adult psychiatric clinic in a medical school hospital, a family agency, a visiting nurse agency, and a State rehabilitation agency. As Coleman points out, the major goals of this project for patients and their families were in many ways closely comparable to those of the new programs being developed in community mental health centers. It is all the more useful, therefore, as the planning for these centers proceeds, to learn from the experiences and understanding gained by this project: It demonstrated not only the value to be derived from community services of one kind or another, and the necessity of their coordination with the hospital for effective use, but also many of the reasons why achieving such coordination is so difficult.

One of the many interesting findings reported by Coleman was that, by and large, the public health nurses' usual routines of operation lent themselves more readily to work with the ex-mental hospital patient than did those of some of the other agency services that were part of the project. It would appear from other experience, as well, that public health nurses can be of particular help in the successful care of psychiatric patients in their own homes, in lieu of hospitalization or to permit early convalescent leave. Through home visits they can provide family counseling, inquire into and observe the welfare of children in the family, spot early signs of trouble, and enlist appropriate help for family members as well as for the index patient. This was substantiated, for instance, in the account by Pasamanick *et al.* in their 1967 "Schizophrenics in the Community: An Experimental Study in the Prevention of Hospitalizations" (10). It was also demonstrated through a pilot project, conducted as part of a community care project at the Columbia Presbyterian Medical Center. Public health nurses with psychiatric consultation and back-up services followed schizophrenic patients, after their discharge from the New York State Psychiatric Institute, and offered services to them and to their families so as to help maintain them in the community and to prevent their further social breakdown. In recognition of the especial importance of measures for the psychological protection of children in such situations, inclusion in this project was limited to patients who were members of a family group. Nurses paid special attention to how the parent's illness affected the children; they tried to fortify family strengths and resources, particularly on behalf of the children, and they mobilized remedial measures from the Medical Center and other community agencies, as indicated.

Drawing on Caplan's "Crisis Model of Mental Health and Disorder," Irvine, in a 1964 article, "Children at Risk," (11) makes a strong case for the inclusion in preventive mental health programs of skilled and, above all, prompt assessments and age-appropriate ways of relieving pathogenic anxieties and confusions, on the part of children who have been exposed to the crisis arising out of the fact that their parents have recently been admitted to a mental hospital.

And so, as evidenced from the foregoing sampling of the literature, there does appear to be at least some expression of concern, documentation of need, and service program approaches to aspects of this problem. However, these have not as yet become *coalesced,* so as to exert a significant influence on practice.

Of course, mechanisms would have to be developed and funding secured in order to carry out measures such as the routine family-focused evaluations recommended above, and those services that Mrs. Ginsburg discusses in Part II of this paper. As we see it, the requisite planning and implementation needs to proceed at governmental levels and in the private as well as public sectors.

It seems extraordinarily timely, therefore, to attempt to insure that this issue, so widely neglected, receive due attention in the current planning of comprehensive community mental health centers, and by the Joint Commission on Mental Health of Children, Inc. *

But more widespread recognition and understanding of the problem seems to be the necessary prerequisite to any reorganiz-

* Since this paper was presented, a Digest of the Commission's Final Report has appeared, and the Report itself, "Crisis of Child Mental Health: Challenge for the 1970's" has been published (Harper & Row, 1970). The crisis needs to which this paper seeks to draw attention are indeed in keeping with the Report's emphasis on prevention, family supports, and high priority for young children.

ing and repatterning of services. Those of us who deal primarily either with adults or with children tend to develop outlooks that are specific to our own particular settings. We need to acquire a greater capacity for "binocular vision," as it were, so that instead of separate images of the sick parent and the young child, these two images can be fused into a view of their *interactions in the total family context.* The crucial variables thereby come to be far more readily apparent, as to whether any or what kind of interrelated preventive and treatment measures are indicated in each specific family situation. Many of us also need to stretch our professional capacity for identification, beyond the settings in which we work and beyond the customary recipients of our direct service.

One's outlook, for example, if one is working in a State hospital, tends to highlight the frustrations and shortcomings that are to be encountered in dealing with local community-based settings. Similarly, from within such community or child care settings, obstacles to one's own work in dealing with hospitals become more clearly evident; thus, hospitals are apt to be viewed, from that vantage point, as remote citadels with which it is unduly hard to communicate. But the current goals of comprehensive community mental health programs—with psychiatric hospitals as a component resource—will in the long run rest on the capacity of professionals to identify with service networks as a whole and with more of the varied segments of the total population being served.

The population segments on which we have focused today are parents with frank mental illness and their young children. As psychiatrists, we have responsibilities toward both. We have sought to draw your attention to the human-ecological aspects of the shift toward community care of the mentally ill. While this promises to reduce the social disability among psychotic parent-patients, the price for such gains could be an increase over time of the psychological disorders of their children. The purpose of this paper is to identify that risk, so that such an outcome may be avoided through appropriate measures.

REFERENCES

1. Goldman, Rose. "Digest of Recent Literature on Children of Mentally Ill Parents." Citizens' Committee for Children of New York, Inc. 1962 (mimeographed).
2. Citizens' Committee for Children of New York, Inc. "Young Children of Mentally Ill Parents," April 1962 (mimeographed).
3. Ekdahl, Miriam C., Rice, Elizabeth P., and Schmidt, William M. "Children of Parents Hospitalized for Mental Illness," *Amer. J. Public Health,* **52,** No. 3, 428-435 (March 1962).
4. Sobel, David E. "Children of Schizophrenic Patients: Preliminary Observations on Early Development." *Am. J. Psychiatry,* **118,** No. 6, 512-517 (December 1961).
5. Rutter, Michael. *Children of Sick Parents, An Environmental and Psychiatric Study*. Maudsley Monograph No. 16 Oxford Univ. Press, London, 1966.
6. Sussex, James N., Gassman, Frances, and Raffel, S. C. "Adjustment of Children with Psychotic Mothers in the Home." *Amer. J. Orthopsychiatry,* **33,** No. 5, 849-854 (October 1963).
7. Higgins, Jerry. "Effects of Child Rearing by Schizophrenic Mothers." *J. Psychiatric Res.* **4,** 153-167 (1966).
8. Rice, Elizabeth P., and Krakow, Sylvia G. "Hospitalization of a Parent for Mental Illness: A Crisis for Children," *Amer. J. Orthopsychiatry,* **36,** No. 5, 868-872 (October 1966).
9. Coleman, Jules V. "A community Project in Behalf of the Hospitalized Mentally Ill Patient: The Cooperative Care Project." *Amer. J. Psychiatry,* **124,** No. 1, 76-79 (July 1967).
10. Pasamanick, Benjamin, Scarpitti, Frank R., and Dinitz, Simon. *Schizophrenics in the Community: An Experimental Study in the Prevention of Hospitalization,* Appleton-Century-Crofts, New York, 1967, pp. 129-132.
11. Irvine, Elizabeth E. "Children at Risk," Case Conference, Vol. 10, 1964. (Also reprinted in *Crisis Intervention: Selected Readings,* Howard J. Pared, ed., Family Association of America, New York, 1964, pp. 220-226.)

Chapter II

Young Children of Mentally Ill Parents: Part II

Ethel L. Ginsburg, A.C.S.W.

Dr. Bernard has outlined the reasons for our longstanding and mounting concern about the young children of mentally ill parents who are the victims of the community's failure to provide the "continuity of care" that is widely endorsed but less widely practiced. This concern is heightened by the continuous stream of professional and popular articles celebrating the "record drop" in the State hospital census, on the apparent assumption that stabilization on drugs in the protected environment of a State hospital will necessarily immunize the patient, especially a woman, against the impact of what awaits her at home. This may, and often does, include poor or no housing; the reestablishment of eligibility for Public Assistance, involving reapplication and reinvestigation; the immediate return of her young children, who may have been farmed out to relatives or placed in temporary shelters when the mother was hospitalized. In some instances, her children are waiting on the doorstep when she arrives.

It would take a strong, stable person to deal with all of this, especially Public Assistance and housing, even without a hastily reassembled family to take care of. When the mother is neither strong nor stable, when she is still psychologically fragile and vulnerable, when her children may still be showing evidence of the fear and anxiety aroused by her bizarre behavior prior to hospitalization, one does not need professional expertise to anticipate trouble, not only for the patient but for her children.

Why, then, has so little attention been paid to what follows brief hospitalization and, too often, precedes readmission? Perhaps this should be amended to read, "Why has so little been done about what is known?"

During most of this decade, the Citizens' Committee for Children of New York has been asking this question of those who were in a position to answer it. The answers go something like this:

> "It certainly is a problem. Of course, many of the readmissions could be prevented if supportive services were available when the patient first comes home, and periodically thereafter, as needed."
>
> "The hospital people don't seem to know that a family exists; they only see the patient as he functions in the hospital and assume that he will carry on even without any help."
>
> "Social agencies don't accept their responsibility for easing the children back into the home, after they've been placed during the mother's absence, and providing supportive services to help them stay at home."
>
> "We don't seem to understand that mental illness is seldom merely an acute episode that will clear up and go away. Even those who should know it best—the doctors in the hospitals—don't do their discharge planning as if they did."

In our efforts to arouse professional interest in these vulnerable children and their equally vulnerable parents, the Citizens' Committee for Children called the meetings that Dr. Bernard mentioned in the preceding section. We gathered case material from a variety of agencies, presented the issues and the problems, and found that, after full and free discussion, there was complete agreement that both patient and family were being severely penalized by the community's failure to provide what it knew was needed and what it knew how to do. That, may I add, was in 1962.

The participants in our 1962 meeting contributed fifty case vignettes, most of which demonstrated the destructive impact on families of the lack of "continuity of care." Among the fifty cases were a few—very few—that demonstrated what could and did happen when family-centered continuity of care did become a reality. In these cases the husband or wife or other close relative of the patient was helped to plan for the care of the children, during the period of hospitalization and in preparation for the patient's return, and supportive services continued until the patient and family were able to carry on unaided. Now, five years later, I wish that funds and staff were available to enable us to follow up these fifty patients, to chart their course and that of their children during this period.

Would we find that the young unmarried mother who was hospitalized during each of her three annual pregnancies has since added four or five new illegitimate babies and hospital readmissions to the national statistics, even though her inability to care for her children was noted five years ago, when they were said to be in jeopardy?

Would we find that the four disturbed, neglected, often-abused children of a paranoid woman are still living with her between her periods of hospitalization, even though at that time and during several preceding years the school and several social agencies reported that "The mother is capable of violence. We fear for the children's safety"?

Or would we find in the few families that did receive continuous support—with psychiatric supervision, homemaker service, day care for the younger children, social services as and when needed, day hospital care for the patient as and when needed—that these families were able to function as families, with the mentally ill parent gradually assuming and carrying the responsibilities that would have been far too heavy to carry alone. The H. family was one of the fortunate few.

The H. Family

Homemaker service was requested because Mrs. H. had been *readmitted* to a State hospital on September 14, 1960.

The family included Mr. H., aged 40, and three children, a boy aged 9 and two girls aged 14 and 2. Mr. H. was employed five days a week, leaving the house at 8:15 and returning about 6. Mr. H. thought that the 14-year-old girl would be able to look after the younger children from 5 until 6 P.M., if the homemaker could come in at about 8 in the morning. Mr. H. said that she was a responsible girl and had often assisted her mother with the care of the younger children. It was arranged that a homemaker would be assigned five days a week from 8:15 A.M. to 5:15 P.M.

The Supervising Field Worker made a home call in late afternoon to talk with Mr. H., who had remained home from work to meet the homemaker, and to introduce her to the children and discuss the routine of the household. He felt that he would be able to look after the children adequately during the hours the homemaker was not on duty and on Saturday and Sunday. It was agreed that the homemaker would assume full responsibility for the care of the children, plan, market, and prepare the meals, bathe the youngest child, and take her out-of-doors to play. Mr. H. would leave a list of needed food items for the homemaker, or any special suggestions he had regarding meals. He also agreed that, with the shopping, cooking, house cleaning, and care of the children, the homemaker might find it difficult to find time to take the laundry to the laundromat, and he thought that he could do this on Saturday morning. The plan was left flexible in the interim, with the understanding that the homemaker would try to wheel the clothes over in a shopping cart if she had the time.

Although the 9-year-old boy was usually self-directing, the homemaker found that on occasion he did not come home after school. When questioned, he said that he visited school friends. This was discussed with Mr. H. and it was agreed that it would be better for R. to come directly home after school, and then go to visit his friends or play. This would make it possible for the homemaker to provide better care and supervision. The eldest girl always came directly home from school and was careful to advise the homemaker when she had other plans.

During the five months before Mrs. H. was discharged from the hospital, both Mr. H. and the children became very much attached to the homemaker and used her services to good advantage. Mr. H. was described by the homemaker as a king, thoughtful man, who took considerable interest in his children. At times he showed worry about his wife's recovery and expressed the hope to the homemaker that she would soon be home and able to carry on, as she did before she went to the hospital.

Early in February 1961, Mr. H. told the homemaker that Mrs. H. was to be released in a few weeks. He wondered whether the homemaker would stay on until Mrs. H. was able to manage alone, and he was given this assurance. Later, the hospital social worker advised the agency worker of plans for Mrs. H's discharge.

When Mrs. H. returned home on February 15, she reported that, when the children had visited her in the hospital, they had expressed warm feelings for the homemaker. She spoke freely about her illness, saying that she knew it would be some time before she would be able to resume all of the home and child care responsibilities. She too was given assurance that we would continue homemaker service until she felt quite able to manage alone, and her doctor felt this was the best plan.

Arrangements had been made for Mrs. H. to attend the aftercare clinic on a regular basis, and the homemaker continued to remain with the family. From the observations of the social worker during her periodic visits from February to April 1961, plus the comments of the homemaker, there was no question but that Mrs. H. continued to use the service well. At the suggestion of the aftercare clinic worker, as relayed to the Homemaker Service Program, the homemaker encouraged Mrs. H. gradually to take greater responsibility for the children and for household management. On April 21, 1961, Homemaker Service was terminated on the recommendation of the psychiatrist at the aftercare clinic, who felt that Mrs. H. was then ready to resume complete responsibility for her home. When this was discussed with Mrs. H., she agreed that she was ready for this.

In recent years, many of us have participated at some length in planning for comprehensive community mental health services in New York State, and in developing plans for the Community Mental Health Centers that will, it is hoped, provide the link that will result in true family-centered continuity of care. But this is still not quite around the corner; it is a hope, not yet a reality. During this decade, we have lost many children and parents who might have been salvaged. We cannot afford to continue to wait for the Community Mental Health Center millennium. The studies and demonstration projects that Dr. Bernard has described point the way to what can be done now. *

It might be well for medical staff members of our psychiatric hospitals—state, county, and municipal—to embark on a round of home visits, so as to see for themselves what it is that their patients are returning to, or coming back from when they are readmitted. I would urge that the round of visits also include the well-baby wards in our municipal hospitals, where the infants who are born out of wedlock to some of these patients wait for placement, often for months, as well as the temporary shelters where youngsters pile up as they wait. We at the Citizen's Committee for Children would be happy to help arrange such visits. We know that people who work in one setting are often unaware of what goes on in another, even though the two may be interrelated, even interdependent. We have found visits an excellent antidote to professional isolation.

To demonstrate that ours is not a new concern, let me quote from "Babies Who Wait," the report of a 1959 Citizens' Committee survey of all boarder babies in general hospitals awaiting foster care placement:

Miss H.

> Miss H. had borne her first child when she was 19, in 1947. Soon thereafter, she was admitted to a municipal hospital, given electric shock treatment, released, and allow-

* Now, as this volume goes to press, community mental health sources are no more plentiful than they were in 1962 and the "revolving-door" policy of brief hospitalization still continues. Whatever its merits for some patients, one result is that infants and young children are popping in and out of foster care at an accelerated pace; and the incidence of parent-patient illness in their families continues to rise.

> ed to return to her mother and child. The following year she was readmitted and later transferred to a State hospital. She was discharged and later readmitted, pregnant with a child who was subsequently placed and is still in foster care. Released once more, Miss H. was out of the hospital for four years; then she was returned, leaving behind her a third child; this one, like the first, was cared for by her mother. Released again, this time after only four months, Miss H. became pregnant again and was soon readmitted to the mental hospital. The fourth baby, the one included in our study, was placed in an institution and later in a boarding-home. She is still there and Miss H., according to the last report, is still in the mental hospital.

Our 1959 report comments as follows:

> There are, of course, limits to current knowledge and skill in psychiatric treatment, and prognosis is always difficult. Yet it would seem that at some earlier point in this not atypical revolving-door history, the mental hospitals which had known Miss H. might have been able to make a more realistic evaluation of the patient's ability to function in the community. Failing such a realistic appraisal, patients continue to be discharged and readmitted on what would appear to be a trial-and-error basis, and children are born to become public charges.

We question society's right to send a fragile, vulnerable, schizophrenic patient out into the world to have another baby each time before she is readmitted to the hospital, and then to compound this injury to her and her numerous progeny by failing to recognize her inability to function and her children's need for protection. Family planning is obviously needed, but reliance on the PILL for these patients would be as unrealistic as today's reliance on the likelihood that they will continue their chemotherapy with any regularity.

As most of you know, in some parts of New York State, tranquilizers are supplied by mail to post-hospital patients who have little or no actual contact with any responsible medical or other representative of the State hospital or of any other institution. In the City of New York, after a token year on the rolls of the State Department of Mental Hygiene Aftercare Clinics, patients are discharged and presumably transferred to the outpatient psychiatric departments of local municipal hospitals. It is no secret that, with few exceptions, this transfer remains a paper transaction and the patient is lost until he reappears for readmission.

Let me make clear here that we are not talking about the intermittent hospitalization that is often indicated in chronic psychiatric illness; this should be easily available when and as needed. What we *are* saying is that, in such illness, every effort must be made to reduce the social pressures on the patient and family, so as to prevent the recurring social crises that now beset these families, particularly the children. We are strongly opposed to the constant readmissions that now occur by default and that will continue, so long as responsibility for comprehensive, family-centered aftercare is nobody's business.

If the time comes when there is, in fact, a Community Mental Health Center to cover each geographical segment of the state, working in direct relationship with the state facility covering its area, the gap may be bridged, not only between hospital and community but between mental health services and all the related health, education, and social services. But this is much more likely to happen if, in the meantime, the State Department of Mental Hygiene, the local Community Mental Health Boards, and the appropriate public and voluntary agencies agree that family-centered continuity of care is, in fact, at least as important as the in-hospital care of patients and, if anything, warrants even greater emphasis in a world that is ostensibly committed to the concept of community services. It is not enough to say that the state institutions will soon become centers for "quick-stop therapeutic care and laboratories for research," with major ongoing service to take place in the community, when we know that what is now going on in most of our communities bears no relationship to this pious hope.

The current State Department of Mental Hygiene leadership in New York City, concerned with some 10,000-12,000 patients a year on convalescent status, is well aware of this. But until *local* health and social services accept these patients—and their families—as full citizens of the *local* community, they will continue to be treated as aliens, subject to deportation. And until psychiatric hospital personnel extend their concern for the patient to include his family, diagnosis and treatment will continue in isolation, and prognosis will not even be an educated guess, because it will not be based on knowledge of the key factors in the patient's home environment.

Is it too much to ask that coordinated mental health and child welfare and other social services be provided for these patients and their families? That comprehensive continuity of care be recognized as something more than psychiatric treatment of the patient alone? That it be based on differential evaluation of the family's strengths and weaknesses, and that the needs of the children be a major consideration in pre- and post-hospital planning for their parents? Is this too much to ask? Our experience to date would seem to indicate that it is. *

This failure to provide for the supportive services needed to protect and promote patient welfare and family stability cannot be defended on any rational grounds—medical, social, or fiscal, not to mention moral. New York State has the necessary manpower and financial resources. Its deployment of these resources must reflect its philosophy of public service. Perhaps it is here that one must look for the answers to our questions.

---

* The Citizens' Committee for Children of New York issued in 1970, a report, "Our Children in New York State Psychiatric Hospitals." Based on a 1969 survey of the State Hospitals serving New York City children, it corroborates the unhappy findings of the Joint Commission on the Mental Health of Children and our own growing concern about the fragmentation of the patient between city and state, between public and voluntary sectors, and between mental health and child welfare services.

Chapter III

Practical Psychiatric Problems Involving Children at the County Level

C. L. Bennett, M.D.

The close interrelationship between County Mental Health Services, Welfare, the family service agencies and the County Departments of Health and Education, and physicians in private practice can be coordinated to benefit children of mentally ill parents. This paper will be largely anecdotal: it will draw freely on actual case histories, and will not attempt to contribute to theoretical considerations.

If we are to derive informational value from the specific cases to be outlined, a knowledge of the county mental health facilities and their administration, as a background for events involving these persons, is mandatory.

Dutchess is a county of 200,000—mixed urban, suburban, and rural—whose population is reasonably stable, from the standpoint of continuous residence. In 1962, the county budget for mental health was $64,000, all of which was used for the maintenance of a psychiatric clinic in Poughkeepsie. The current budget, five years later, is $320,000, and 97% of this amount is devoted to supplying increased outpatient community services, only 3% going for inpatient care in a general hospital psychiatric section. In this five-year period, we have initiated a very active child guidance clinic, an alcoholism clinic, rehabilitative services for the mentally retarded and psychiatrically disabled, full-time psychological and social services for the Family Court, an inpatient general hospital service for acute treatment of selected patients; by the end of 1968, we will have our own 2½ million dollar Community

Mental Health Center, to house these outpatient facilities under one roof. The planning for this Center, over a two-year period, required many joint meetings of key personnel from all these facilities and agencies with the Director of County Mental Health Services, members of the County Mental Health Board, and state officials from the Department of Mental Hygiene, who were involved with the projected Center. Communication and coordination between agencies with respect to individual patients had always been good; but these meetings further cemented relationships, the Director serving as a common denominator. The full cooperation of the State Hospital, and its 400-bed decentralized unit devoted entirely to Dutchess, has been assured over the past five years by the fact that the Director of this county inpatient and day care service in the State Hospital is also the appointed Director of Mental Health Services for the county, thus providing a degree of continuity of care, follow-up, and interagency cooperation from full hospitalization, through day care, and out to community facilities that is relatively rare. Further cooperation between State Hospital and community is enhanced by the fact that the Director of the parent hospital (Hudson River) is also a member of the nine-man Community Mental Health Board, which is responsible to county and state for the supervision of all mental health facilities in the county that are supported by public funds.

It is chiefly this underlying framework that has made it possible to cut corners, avoid the disastrous obstructive effects of antagonisms between professional primadonnas, and achieve a degree of cooperation that has made Dutchess a center for research studies on the part of the Milbank Foundation, Columbia University, and the Department of Mental Hygiene, which is considerably interested in coordinating the State Hospital services with newly emerging community resources. This administrative framework also promotes a considerable degree of personal contact between mental health and county government, judiciary, commissioners of Health, Education, and Welfare, family service agencies, and private practitioners which has relevance to individual cases, as I shall try to illustrate.

Case 1

Mrs. S., age 32, resident of Hyde Park, had been admitted twice in six years to the Dutchess Unit for relatively acute episodes of catatonic schizophrenia, with the usual periods of partial remission characteristic of that illness. She had a two-year-old child and the neighbors complained to Welfare that the child was malnourished, not receiving proper nutrition, and neglected. The husband of Mrs. S. was large and hostile and the neighbors were not about to sign a formal complaint; without it, Welfare was reluctant to act. The Welfare Commissioner, knowing that Mrs. S. had formerly been our patient, conferred with us about the impasse.

Since Mrs. S. had been formally discharged three years previously, the hospital could not take action to return her, but the County Director of Mental Health services could investigate. He called the Health Commissioner and asked that a specific public health nurse, who had visited the home after Mrs. S. had returned from the hospital with the baby two years before and was welcome in the home, be asked to revisit and report her opinion about the child's condition. Her report was sufficiently alarming for us to delegate one of our staff psychiatrists, who had cared for Mrs. S. on a previous admission and who was currently doing pre-care and follow-up duties, in addition to his inpatient responsibilities, to visit the next day, with the public health nurse to help pave the way.

He spent an hour in the home, and observed the feeding; it was completely inadequate and punctuated by sharp arguments, in which the mother vainly tried to defend her ideas against a concerted, and completely ignorant, tirade about feeding put forth by her husband and his 80-year-old mother. The visiting physician found that this was a daily occurrence, that the mother always lost, and that the child was indeed suffering from malnutrition, as well as from the constantly hostile atmosphere in the home.

All three agencies then combined forces, after mutual consultation, to induce the family to take the child to the office of a local pediatrician, who was briefed ahead of time by Mental Health. This individual, a friend of twenty years standing, put on a performance that, under other circumstances, would have earned him an Oscar. After examining the child, he announced that she was "dying of starvation"; he literally roared at the parents that, unless they took the child immediately for admission to the pediatric service at Vassar Hospital, he would personally sign criminal charges against them for neglect, and as prearranged by telephone consultation, he dispatched his office nurse to lead them to the hospital by car, so as to insure compliance.

Relieved of this responsibility, the mother promptly readmitted herself to the hospital, "to get away from home and get my nerves back." The child regained normal weight in four weeks and was returned home at the same time that the mother was released from hospital, following several hours spent in the model kitchen of the ward getting instruction in nutrition. She also returned home to an altered situation, in that she was now on convalescent care and was visited weekly by both our social service and the public health nurse, as one of the 10% of released patients we share responsibility for with Public Health. Periodic examinations are carried out at the pediatric clinic, and for the past two years the father and mother-in-law have not again attempted to manage the situation.

Case 2

Mrs. B., age 33, had never been hospitalized, but had been for three months under the care of a psychoanalyst, who subsequently informed us that she had been developing a deepening depression, had not appeared for the last three appointments at his office, and had rejected his efforts to get her to return. She was undergoing a trial separation from her husband, a highly trained program analyst for I.B.M., and Family Court had temporarily given her custody of the three children, ages 4, 8, and 12. Early one morning, about a year ago, she collected all of the various types of sedative medication in the house, prepared a species of barbiturate soup in warm milk, and divided it between the children, informing them that it was a "new kind of vitamin." With that accomplished, she retired to her own bedroom and took about 120 tablets of Equanil that she had been accumulating for months.

Fortunately, the estranged husband, sensing his wife's illness and potential, made it a habit to check daily on the home at the time when the children normally left for school. When they did not appear, he called the police, entered the home, and found all four in coma. Two of the children recovered quickly; the third developed a hypostatic pneumonia but recovered without complication. The mother remained comatose for 48 hours and, on regaining consciousness, was extremely depressed, delusional, and totally without insight. After about ten weeks in the only locked ward in the 5,000-bed hospital, she was reviewed by a release committee of three experienced psychiatrists and adjudged ready to be transferred to the open Dutchess County Unit.

At that point, a full hour's conference was held with the Family Court Judge in his chambers, and it was determined to review the conditions of the separation agreement by another court hearing before the patient was formally released from the hospital. This was done: The court decision regarding supervision of the children was reversed, and the patient directed to attend the Day Care Center for a period of six months. This period completed, the case was again reviewed by Family Court, in conjunction with both psychiatric and psychological consultation on a county level, and she was "graduated" to returning to her business position and to attending the outpatient clinic once weekly for another six months. When last reviewed, the patient had achieved a moderate amount of insight, and there was a possibility of reorganizing the marriage, with continuing therapeutic support. It may be noted that this was a matter of locking the barn door after the horse was *almost* stolen; but it should also be noted that the whole dismal sequence took place before hospitalization became mandatory, before it was even brought to the attention of physicians in public practice.

I shall be as brief as possible in outlining the last case, chosen because it again illustrates the importance of intercommunication and cooperation between diversified public agencies.

Case 3

This case involved a 40-year-old married woman in the southern tier of the county, who had never been hospitalized or even treated psychiatrically as an outpatient. The first referral came from a professional friend of long standing, the Director of the Castle Point V.A. Hospital in Dutchess, who wanted to find out if anything could be done to relieve him of daily visits from the wife of one of his tuberculosis patients, who was adamant about the immediate release of her husband "because there is no reason why he shouldn't be working to support me and the two children." The husband ran a daily P.M. temperature, had bilateral cavitation, a positive sputum, and worked as a short-order cook. None of these factors meant anything to the wife, and on one occasion she had succeeded in getting her husband out of bed and outside the building in his hospital gown before being apprehended.

While we were pondering whether there was anything that we could legally do to help Castle Point, another call came through from Public Health on the same person, stating that she had refused to allow her two teen-aged boys to visit the County Health Clinic for chest X-rays, "because they would probably pick up tuberculosis in a place like that." Persistent efforts on the part of public health nurses were unsuccessful, largely because of the boys, aged 14 and 16, who were well known to the Children's Court, where the court psychologist had decided that they were "totally without parental guidance or identification," and to the County Psychiatric clinic, where a social worker had described them, in desperate frustration, as "black-leather-jacketed hoodlums, headed for reform school."

The seriousness of the situation, in regard to community public health, led to consultation with the Health Commissioner, and it was decided that Mental Health would attempt to alleviate the situation by direct involvement of the County Judge, if he would agree. He pointed out that he had no real jurisdiction in the matter and could not order the principals to appear before him, but that he would be glad to bring the influence of the court to bear, if they were brought to him on a regular appoint-

> ment by the County Health Department. This was arranged by the Health Commissioner; but shortly after a definite appointment was made with the Judge, the boys appeared at the clinic for X-rays, and the mother informed Castle Point that she had "changed her mind" about influencing her husband to leave the hospital.

This particular case was not, basically, a psychiatric problem, but it is cited to illustrate what can be accomplished by the coordination and utilization of various county services to accomplish an obviously necessary end.

By way of summary and conclusions, I would like to make a few admittedly generalized statements, for purposes of discussion, that are not easily subject to either research or proof:

1. Obviously no person in a responsible position, who has the emotional well-being of children in mind, is entitled to minimize the potentially disastrous effects of exposing them to psychotic parents. The current trend toward open hospitals, prompt treatment, and early release to the community, as opposed to protracted hospitalization, in an effort to minimize the "social breakdown syndrome," will certainly increase the frequency of this problem during the next decade. However, in maintaining perspective on this thorny problem, it is probable that, in the definite majority of cases wherein disabling emotional pressures are being exerted on children, neither parent has ever been hospitalized, is psychotic, or even is certifiable for admission or retention in a state-licensed hospital. It would seem indicated that a strong and concerted effort toward increasing the awareness of this problem among those in closest contact with the public, such as the clergy, family service agencies, public health nurses, and general practitioners, might have the best chance of effecting prevention. This might be done best by enlisting the services of the Mental Health Societies, at county and state level, as a part of their information and education programs.

2. From the standpoint of hospitalized patients, certain precautions are routinely observed here, and are suggested for consideration.

A. Where in-hospital psychiatric and psychological study of a parent indicates potential physical or emotional threat to young children, the return to community is determined formally, written up, and signed by a Release Committee of three experienced psychiatrists, and then passed upon by review of the Hospital Director.

B. In cases where the courts have been involved, we do not hesitate to make recommendations regarding the placement of limiting factors on the offending parent. In a substantial number of these cases, separation or divorce is already pending. Where the question of firearms is involved, which is not infrequent in Dutchess County, both the family and the Sheriff's Office are informed of the advisability of removing them from the home.

C. Where there is evidence that children are already adversely affected, every effort is made to induce the family to initiate treatment in the form of family therapy in our own Day Care Center, or in the extensive program undertaken at the Astor Home Child Guidance Center. It is surprising how often the families and patient will recognize and accept the necessity of carrying out this joint attack.

D. We have found, after release of a patient on convalescent care, that welfare social service, the public health nurses, family service agencies, and even private practitioners have been more helpful in coordinating with our own psychiatric staff and social service to help in alleviating potential harm.

E. Whenever possible, we arrange return visits to our own outpatient clinic, to enable family members (including older children) to be interviewed in addition to the patient.

F. Finally, while it is incumbent upon us to do everything that we can from the standpoint of adult psychiatric supervision, whether inpatient, partial hospitalization, or follow-up care in the community, the questions of *what* specific harm is being done to the child, *how* it is being done, and *what* to do about it still lie properly in the realm of child psychiatry. Unfortunately, expert service and consultation in this field, which is crucial to the problem at hand, is almost impossible to obtain outside metropolitan areas. We have two Board-certified child psychiatrists for a population of 200,000; they are already completely involved in civic responsibilities to education, rehabilitation of the retarded, clinic work, and consultation to the Family Court, in addition to their in-patient responsibilities, so that significant involvement in this field is impossible. As a result, decisions involving diagnosis, treatment, and disposition of children are being made by persons of limited experience, and with almost no qualifications in this highly specialized field.

Section 2

Parents under Unmanageable Stress

Introduction

In Chapter IV of this section, Lillian C. Lampkin, Assistant Professor at the Hunter College School of Social Work, hits us between the eyes with a well-documented report of the *reality* of children and families living in lower-class neighborhoods—particularly those where Puerto Ricans and Negroes predominate. She stresses the fact that parents often accept events—resign themselves to them—even though they would prefer what middle-class standards dictate. She emphasizes what we already know but often disregard—namely, that peer group pressure is extremely powerful. She reiterates the widely held opinion that our public schoools—as much of an establishment as many of the factories where these children will later seek employment—have created an environment too foreign to the slum and ghetto homes and neighborhoods for them to adapt to. And she ends by challenging us to exert pressure for major social changes.

Miss Elizabeth Elmer brings a new contribution from the Infant Accident Study, Children's Hospital, Pittsburgh. She is one of the people who first called attention to what has come to be known as the "battered-child syndrome." Special legislation has been enacted recently in many states for the protection of these children. The paper included here is particularly pertinent to the subject matter of this monograph. Miss Elmer brings us findings from a follow-up study of twenty-two abused children, a study that focused not only on the victims but also on the mothers, for it was in almost all cases the mother who was responsible for the abuse. The findings here reported shed light on the relentless stresses that bore down on mothers who finally—sometimes repeatedly—lost control sufficiently to resort to this degree of violence. The paper ends with a plea for preventive measures and again for social change.

Chapter VI concerns itself with the problem of multiple, at times compulsive, pregnancies. It seeks to understand the tie between deprived, often harrassed and depressed, mothers and their neglected children. It raises the question, since many of these mothers had themselves been separated from their families and placed during childhood, of whether placement of neglected children of deprived mothers is the best way of dealing with them, and outlines a program designed to complement the mother's child-rearing task. Finally, it calls attention to the neglected child turned delinquent, who receives little or no care, and suggests an administrative reform at the state level.

Chapter IV

Alienation as a Coping Mechanism

"Out Where the Action Is"

Lillian C. Lampkin, M.S.W.

There is no intent, in the subtitle to my remarks, to be frivolous. Rather it is a serious effort to direct your attention away from the inner dynamics of personality and family relations toward the outer demands and rewards of the social situation, the stresses and strains created by social institutions, and the consequences of membership in the underclass. I see my role here today as sharing with you some of what I have learned through my experiences in the marketplace.

Let me say frankly that my experience compels a view of alienations—as well as of acting-out—that may not be traditional. I think that what we call "deviant" and "acting out" may represent a meaningful and conforming adaptation to many an individual's reality. In a neighborhood where people believe that the world is made up of "smart guys" and "suckers," where aggression within families and between neighbors and the police, the investigator, or other representatives of the larger society is commonplace, gang fights are not surprising. In a neighborhood where the impulse toward a decent home, a decent job or just a good suit of clothes is continually blocked, where status is attained by being cool, hard, and tough—in such a neighborhood, stealing, conning the teachers, and dropping out of school are what your peers expect of you.

I met Pedro at a community center in just such a neighborhood. He was 19, had graduated from high school cum laude, but had never worked. He was a brown Puerto Rican and this was during a period of recession. Witty and moody, he could burst into violent anger at an imagined insult. I saw him slap a girl so hard her lip bled because he thought she was laughing at him. I recall him pacing my office like a caged tiger, imploring me to agree that "It's not what you know, but who you know that counts in this stinking world." But I also remember his gentle kindness to me, when my desk clock was stolen; how he tried to get it back and consoled me when I cried. He said it was good to be able to cry sometimes; he hadn't cried since he was five. In this light, the "acting out" behavior of adolescents represents both a high degree of socialization within the context of a real life situation and conformity to norms and values that have been legitimized in a given social circle.

In similar fashion, what many of us characterize as "alienation" does not—I think—result so much from rejection of majority values or culture, but from the acceptance of pressing realities of underclass life in an affluent society. Two examples come to mind: At a small city agency set up to work with multi-problem families, a group of unmarried mothers in their late twenties was formed. When one young lady arrived early for the first meeting, my assistant went out to chat with her, while awaiting the arrival of the other women. After the group started, my assistant returned to the offiice and said, "I've got news for you. Miss Jay would give her little finger for a wedding ring, but she knows that she'll never get one."

A group of older parents asked for a speaker to discuss discipline of adolescents. A social worker who had many years experience with adolescents in low income neighborhoods was secured. Eventually the discussion got around to dating, intercourse, and pregnancy. The social worker was shocked to discover that the women were not asking her how they could help their daughters avoid out-of-wedlock pregnancies, but how they could postpone them for a year or two. To these women pregnancy before, and generally without, marriage was an accepted, inevitable part of life. As a matter of fact, some of our teenage girls sought pregnancy. This they thought—or rather, they fancied—would be a way of escape from intolerable homes.

The reactions of these women point clearly to one of the mistakes we so frequently make. We confuse what is accepted with what is valued. Miss Jay would have loved marriage, its ceremony and symbols; the older women were not eager for illegitimate grandchildren. They knew what the larger society believed about out-of-wedlock pregnancy and illegitimacy, and they were even in sympathy with the values on which these beliefs were based. But all had come to terms with the realities of their existence. Were these women atypical? I do not think so. A group of families served by the agency were studied in depth. The researchers found

> no evidence that these women reject or are ignorant of the central values of American culture. They all subscribe, at least verbally, to the importance of education, have higher hopes for their children, and want a higher plane of living.

Why then did they fail so miserably in moving toward these aspirations? Here we come face to face with what it means to be black, poor, and ghettoed in rich, white America. How many of us know what it is like to live in dilapidated, congested houses, unfit for human habitation? Are we acquainted with the lack of teaching or the crushing impact of "the system" in slum schools? Have we confronted the erosion of unemployment?

Only when we do confront such conditions and grasp their impact, only then will we realize the overwhelming inevitability of the women's failure. Only then can we begin to understand why they think and behave as they do.

Recently at a conference on the racial crisis in America today, I met a brilliant and bitter young Negro man. In trying to explain himself—and poor Negroes in general—to his fellow delegates, most of whom were middle-class and white, he told how he had gone for weeks without a good night's sleep because he had to stay alert, lest the necessity to ward off an attack by hungry rats arise. He then went on to describe how being tired and tense influenced his performance on his job and eventually got him fired.

Our women had little of this insight. But more important to their functioning than lack of insight was their lack of knowledge about the social systems and institutions that were central to their lives. Less than a third of the respondents in the study mentioned above had any specific perception of how the welfare budget is conceived. Two-thirds thought the regular check was supposed to cover all their needs, "including *all* clothing, medical expenses and household goods." Many had heard of people getting extra things, but "few of them realized that the possibility of receiving nonrecurring allotments from the Department of Welfare was built into the system and rightfully theirs, rather than whim or favor from a particular social investigator." (1)

They were equally ignorant of the educational system. One mother, when asked how long her children should remain in school, thought for a while and said that they should graduate from grammar school because this would help with a job. Since the interviewer knew better, she probed further, asking "Suppose this doesn't work?" The mother thought again and responded that then they would have to go to college—without any notion of the sequential nature of education, of the fact that high school comes between grammar school and college. In fact, they had little knowledge about the interrelationship between education and jobs—either with respect to amount or kind. And so it was with many other areas of living.

However, because education is so crucial to success in a world of expanding technology, I want to discuss the school briefly. In *Youth in the Ghetto: A Study of the Consequences of Powerlessness,* the authors say:

> An appraisal of education in Central Harlem leads to the conclusion that the schools have lost faith in the ability of their pupils to learn, and the community had lost faith in the ability of the schools to teach. (2)

One of the adolescents interviewed in the course of this very extensive study commented that "the kids is smart. They get out before they become blooming idiots." Our experience in

Central Harlem attested to this boy's wisdom. In reviewing school records, we found time and time again constantly deteriorating performance, beginning especially in the third year and continuing throughout the period of school attendance. Recently I have been exposed to what are perceived as radical new ideas in early childhood education. They call for structure and direct teaching in both the nursery and kindergarten, on the assumption that, for the lower-class child, the battle of learning is lost before the child enters school.

Even if this is not so, our children found the school inhospitable—to them and to their family's life style. It was a place where they had difficulty communicating; a situation that seemed to demand that they renunciate their uniqueness. Edgar Friedenberg in his book *The Vanishing Adolescent* calls attention to the impact of social status on the total school experience, and the depressing fate of the lower-class student within the educational system. Friedenberg says: "All aspects of a youngster's life in High School—not only his social life outside the classroom—are strongly influenced by his family's social status". (3) This and other studies seem to indicate that, regardless of native endowment, the students with higher social status consistently receive the best grades. Moreover, when it comes to extracurricular activities, they also receive the offices, the acclaim and other privileges and rewards. Clearly, the school is not an effective instrument of either education or socialization for the lower-class child.

However, it is not only his school, but also his neighborhood that lacks the appropriate ingredients for social nurture. Day in and day out, these young people see their older brothers, uncles, and other idle men hanging around on street corners. For many, the only men they know who have "bread" in their pockets, a good suit on their backs, and a car are the numbers runner and the "pusher." Youngsters living in black slums can grow up without ever seeing the "man of the house" get up in the morning to go to work or come home at night. In such a situation, confused, overwhelmed, unaware parents are unable to resist the pull of the streets on their children.

During the 1964 riots in Harlem, I asked our 15-year-old

messenger if he had been involved. He said no, not yet; but his friends had. To my "Good Lord, don't they know that they can be killed?" he replied "So what!" Seeing nothing much in the present or on the horizon to live for, they viewed death with indifference. As the authors of the proposal for Mobilization for Youth point out:

> The major problem in dealing with self-defeating adaptations is that they generally become "functionally autonomous"—that is, once they come into existence, they tend to persist, quite independent of the forces to which they were originally a response.

The other side of this coin is the growing tendency of many poor minority group youth to view violence and attack as an expression of manhood. They seem to say, "I've been beaten long enough. Now I'm taking over. If nothing else, my aggression asserts that I am."

A colleague told me about a young Puerto Rican college student, a counsellor in camp, who had been on leave during the disturbances in East Harlem. Upon return to camp, this upward-striving young man told shamefacedly about walking down Third Avenue and suddenly finding that he was throwing a bottle. And he said, "You know, it felt good!" Even my middle-class godson finds this mood invigorating; he leaves his home and neighborhood to go play basketball in the slums "because it feels good!"

What I am suggesting is that, if we want to stem the tide of the crisis in disorganization among underclass families, we must address ourselves not simply to the family but to the social conditions in which the family lives. More than in any other social strata, social institutions are crucial to underclass families. Their lives are dominated by them, and they and their children are dependent on them for social nurture. Many of these institutions were designed for another day and another group. Institutional arrangements are haphazard, and their services are focused more on illness than on health. At a recent symposium on troubled children held at Arden House many questions were raised about the character and quality of child welfare services. One is particularly pertinent to our discussion here this morning—namely:

> Are we building resources at the bottom of the hill to catch children after they fall, instead of building fences at the top of the hill so children won't fall in the first place?

Rearrangement and reformation of services and institutions will require radical creative social engineering. If we are to move from our present "patchwork quilt" to a more rational arrangement and delivery of services, we must make courageous decisions about social and economic policies. Dr. Mencher, in the July 1967 issue of *Social Work,* discusses ideological issues that influence the nature of socioeconomic decision-making and affect the direction of change in society. He believes that distribution of income, use of the national income, provision of roles and opportunities for dignified living, and planning and intervention for maximum individual freedom are fundamental ideological issues, which the helping professions must confront and about which they must take a position. He challenges the social professions with these words: "The ideals previously designated as utopian are within realistic reach if we are ready to think in terms of major reforms in society rather than piecemeal programs." It is not enough, he says, simply to place "the disadvantaged on the rungs of the ladder to success." It is the ladder that requires re-evaluation, as well as the functioning of the well-to-do and of their less fortunate neighbors.

For example, how can the affluent suburbanite who earns his money in the city be influenced to take responsibility for solving the problems of the city? Dr. Eli Ginsburg, at the symposium mentioned above, said:

> The notion that the affluent part of the population can come into the city by day, make a good living, and run away from the city at night and live in secluded suburbs free from and uncontaminated by the problem people and all the problems a city

> attracts, and creates and holds is an untenable position.

Dr. Mencher closed his article by suggesting that this problem is a long-standing fundamental controversy that is still with us. In spite of a growing body of legislation, our social policy seems in many ways to be still rooted in the Elizabethan Poor Laws. A review of recent discussions in Congress will, I think, support such a contention. Even the so-called War on Poverty is a guerrilla action, which jumps from brush fire, while viewing the "poor" as all suffering from the same disease and as a blight on our affluent society.

Jerome B. Wiesner in a *New York Times* supplement in April of 1966, said:

> We are living during one of history's most exciting periods —a dynamic time when man has almost limitless choices for good and for evil. We can make any kind of a world that man can agree upon, and if we don't learn to agree a bit better man's days upon this planet may be numbered. I believe that this quarter-century is likely to be the most decisive of any in man's history, for we are undergoing a test unlike any challenge man has ever faced before.

He was addressing himself primarily to problems arising out of advanced technology. I believe that his words apply equally to our crisis in human relations.

To pass the test, we need a knowing, gutsy commitment.

REFERENCES

1. Gordon, Joan. *Poor of Harlem: Social Functioning in the Underclass.* Report to the Welfare Administration, U.S.A. (Welfare Administration Project, 105), Interdepartmental Neighborhood Service Center, New York City, 1965.
2. Harlem Youth Opportunities Unlimited Inc. *Youth in the Ghetto: A Study of the Consequences of Powerlessness and a Blueprint for Change.* New York, 1964.
3. Freidenberg, Edgar Z. *The Vanishing Adolescent.* Dell Publishing Co., New York, 1964.

Chapter V

Child Abuse: A Symptom of Family Crisis *

Elizabeth Elmer, M.S.S.

About ten years ago, a shocking but instructive event came my way: within the brief span of seven days, six infants were admitted to Children's Hospital of Pittsburgh, all with injuries suggesting abuse. All were less than sixteen months of age; and they were admitted in the middle of the night, by exceptionally young parents who gave bizarre histories before melting away. The event taught the obvious lesson that the mistreatment of a child is not a unique case but represents a whole class of child care. As such, it should be possible to study groups of similar cases and to distinguish characteristics of the families and the children. From this conviction grew our study of neglected and abused children and their families, known as the "Fifty Families Study."

One can conceptualize abuse as having a number of determinants—for example, the value system bearing on the worth of children, or the dominant needs and defenses of the abuser. While these and other factors are indeed important, I should like here to focus on the kinds of stress found in the abusive families we have studied.

The "Fifty Families Study" was a retrospective evaluation of children who had been treated at Children's Hospital of Pittsburgh because of multiple skeletal injuries (1). Radiologic

* This paper is based on the study, "Neglected and Abused Children and Their Families," which was supported by the U.S. Public Health Service, National Institute of Mental Health, Grant No. MH 14739.

examination showed that the bone injuries were in different stages of healing and had thus been incurred at different times. Such injuries have been recognized as suggestive of abuse (2, 3), and the young patients have come to be known as "battered babies." Our study group comprised all the fifty patients with this condition who had been seen at Children's Hospital over a thirteen-year period, 1949 to 1962. The majority were under ten months of age when their injuries were identified. In addition to evaluating the current status of the children, we planned to study their caretakers.

All the families were located, but nineteen children could not be seen. The families of six children refused to participate in the study; five other children had been admitted to state institutions for the retarded, and eight children had died—facts that increased our concern for the remaining children. We were able to evaluate thirty-one of the original fifty children, plus two siblings with a history of physical abuse. The children underwent a series of outpatient procedures, designed to assess their physical health, mental functioning, and social adjustment. With respect to four children, we found other explanations for the old injuries and concluded that these children had not been mistreated. The cause of the injuries of seven children could not be determined; but the remaining twenty-two children, on the basis of all available data, were judged to have been abused. In most instances, the agent was thought to be the mother.

Our examinations revealed many difficulties among all the children; but it was the abused group that had the largest proportion of problems of the most serious kind (4). In addition to several instances of retarded growth, half of the group were mentally retarded; many had personality disturbances; and several had permanent handicaps resulting from their old injuries. In view of the state of these children, it seems particularly important to understand the context in which abuse occurs, and on that basis to plan preventive and remedial measures.

At the time of evaluation, a number of the abused children were living with foster families, where they had been placed by the courts following their abusive injuries. Thus it was possible to compare abusive with non-abusive families. The mothers were studied by means of two structured interviews, which yielded data about interpersonal relationships and the day-by-day functioning of the family, as well as information about the child. Each mother also responded to two standardized questionnaires, the Parental Attitude Research Instrument of Schaefer and Bell (5) and the Srole Anomie Scale (6). Social and legal agencies provided data that were important for verification and elaboration of the interview material.

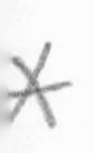

We gathered information on six variables: marital difficulty; household disorganization; personality problems in the mother; negativism toward the child; diversity of punishments; and mother's lack of associations outside the home. On every variable considered, the abusive mothers as a group showed a greater degree of dysfunction than the non-abusive mothers. Three of the variables will be discussed, in order to illustrate important differences.

Marital dissension, although common among both groups, was more overt among the abusive families, as measured by frequency of quarreling, repeated separations and reconciliations, and desertion. Heavy drinking by the fathers was reported by several abusive, but none of the non-abusive mothers. Half of the abusive, but none of the non-abusive mothers said they were afraid of the fathers, and in some instances our collateral data gave ample reason for the mothers' fears. For example, one father who was feared by the mother was in prison following his conviction for murder.

In the area of personality, over half the mothers in both groups were depressed, but there was a contrast in the manner of expressing this feeling: The abusive mothers reported disturbances in eating and sleeping, and a tendency to crying spells, while the non-abusive mothers described little behavior of this kind. Three abusive, but no non-abusive mothers admitted uncontrollable actions in the past. One woman said she probably would have killed another person in a physical battle had someone not intervened.

The most striking difference between the two groups was in the extent of associations outside the home. The abusive mothers belonged to few groups, such as church, PTA, a lodge, or a union, and had almost no close friends who might be companions or sources of help. Our impression was that it was the women themselves who resisted becoming involved in relationships, even when they might have done so. The same isolation was reflected in the absence of ties between the abusive mothers and members of the extended family. The majority stated that no adult on either side of the family could be depended on for help, should the need arise, while all the non-abusive mothers had someone in the extended family to depend on.

In summary, the majority of the families, both abusive and non-abusive, were members of the lower social class, and therefore subject to the stresses of inadequate education, low-paid and insecure work, and lack of material resources. A number of other stressful conditions were more pronounced in the abusive than in the non-abusive group; our results were supported by the comparative scores of the two groups on the pertinent PARI scales and the Srole Anomie Scale (1). I have mentioned, in particular, marital difficulties, emotional problems in the mothers, and absence of associations outside the home. Presumably, although we measured these characteristics at one point in time, the differences between abusive and non-abusive families may be considered stable. However, we were interested in additional criteria that might explain why abuse had occurred at a particular time in the past.

The question of course could not be answered through direct interviews, because of the retrospective nature of the study. Instead we inspected documented facts related to family structure, such as age of mother, number of children, interval between births, and timing of pregnancies—all in relation to the period of hospital treatment of our patient. In this portion of the study, we collected data for abusive, non-abusive, and unclassified families who were caring for the child when the injuries occurred; we eliminated the substitute parents, because they were not then associated with the child.

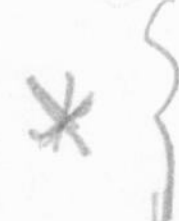

We developed a composite stress score, related to the time of hospital treatment of the patient; it was based on these items, each assigned an arbitrary score of one: (1) three or more children in the family; (2) mother less than 21 years of age; (3) study child conceived out of wedlock; (4) less than one year between births; and (5) mother either pregnant at time of admission of study child, or had borne a child other than the patient during the preceding year. Broad differences between the groups were well defined. Nine of the twenty abusive, but none of the non-abusive or unclassified families had stress scores of three or more. Most strongly associated with abuse was a recent or present pregnancy: Nine of the abusive mothers were pregnant at the time of the patient's hospitalization, and three others had been pregnant within the year previous. In only one of the non-abusive and unclassified families, taken together, was there a similar association of pregnancy and hospitalization of the patient. The difference between the two groups on this variable was significant at the .02 level. *

Still another meaningful fact emerged from examination of pregnancy and birth data. More than 30% of all the children studied were premature by birth weight, a much higher proportion than the national average of 8% (7). Five of the premature babies who were later abused were born to families whose stress scores were three or more, thus adding the shock of premature delivery and the care of an unusually small infant to the already acute problems in the family.

These data show a clear association in our study between child abuse and burdens intimately related to pregnancy and the spacing of children. In addition, they give rise to important questions—for example, what is the meaning of childbirth to these families? If the advent of a child is indeed a critical factor in the abuse of infants, why is the family's distress expressed in such an unacceptable manner?

One of the puzzling aspects of stress research in general is the highly individualized appraisal and response with respect to potentially stressful stimuli. Lazarus believes that four important factors affect appraisal and coping (8): degree of

---

* Chi-square with Yates correction for small numbers. $\chi^2 = 5.61$, $df = 1$, $p = < .02$.

threat of the stimulus; the location and power of the agent of harm; the possibility of alternative actions; and the social or situational constraints influencing the choice of reactions.

With these factors in mind, a hypothetical reconstruction of abuse in our families might go this way: From the nature and intensity of the reaction—namely, repeated assault against the child—we may infer that pregnancy represents a substantial threat to these mothers. Plausible explanations include: the number of babies already born; the brief interval between births, leading to depletion of the mothers' adaptive capacity; and the absence of gratification and support in the marriage. Added to this may well be a sense of being trapped, and a feeling of helplessness because there is no way out. The mother's anxiety would normally be expressed to the father, but here the marital relationship is marked by tension, sometimes fear, and therefore the communication of negative feelings might be difficult or dangerous. It thus becomes necessary for the mother to find some other means of expressing herself.

What other ways are open to her? Cut off as she is from possible relationships in both the extended family and the community, no opportunity exists to ventilate anxiety or to obtain the kind of support that is available to many pregnant women. Furthermore, society requires that pregnancy be welcomed and infants loved, regardless of the mother's feelings or the baby's demands. To the extent that a mother has absorbed this standard, it is doubtful that she can pemit herself to become fully aware of her explosive feelings; instead, she strikes out in response to minute provocations.

In the "Fifty Families Study," child abuse seemed to occur as a reaction to a particularly threatening stimulus—pregnancy—as it impinged on a family already precariously balanced because of multiple stresses in everyday living, personality problems in the mothers, and the absence of meaningful associations both outside and inside the immediate family. * The findings are based on a small number of chil-

* A negative relationship with the child at the time of abuse is also hypothesized but could not be assessed in this study.

dren, all treated in a hospital because of serious injuries; these may not be representative of other populations of abused children and their families. Nevertheless, the speculation may be ventured that the majority of abusive actions occur within the context of stress involving particular difficulty in personal relationships both inside and outside the family and are performed by individuals with few sources of emotional support.

Remedial measures are difficult; they may involve the separation of the child from his family in order to protect him from serious injury or death. Obviously, such drastic treatment does nothing to alter the unhealthy relationships within the family, and it may even lead to the abuse of another child. Prevention is the more hopeful direction. Help during the child-bearing years might be provided by family allowances, as in most other civilized countries. This is one way of lessening everyday burdens and making room for the solution of other complex problems. Particularly vulnerable mothers might be identified through the prenatal clinic or the lying-in hospital; supportive measures and anticipatory guidance would be most meaningful during the pregnancy and neonatal period. Information about family planning needs to be available and clearly understood. Day care centers for infants might permit the mother some respite from the routines of child care.

One could in fact think of a number of measures that would ease the lot of most young families, and that might incidentally have the effect of helping to prevent the abuse of infants and young children. This is indeed the approach that we believe holds the most promise and needs the greatest emphasis.

REFERENCES

1. For a detailed report of the study, see Elmer, E. *Children in Jeopardy,* Univ. Pittsburgh Press, Pittsburgh, 1967.
2. Kempe, C. H., Silverman, F. N., Steele, B. F., Droegemueller, W., and Silver, H. K., "The Battered-child Syndrome," *J.A.M.A.,* **181,** 17-21 (1962).
3. Silverman, F. N. "The Roentgen Manifestations of Unrecognized Skeletal Trauma in Infants." *Amer. J. Roentgenol,* **69,** 413-427 (1953).

4. Elmer, F. and Gregg, G. "Developmental Characteristics of Abused Children." *Pediatrics,* **40,** 596-602 (October, 1967).
5. Schaefer, E. S., and Bell, R. Q. "Development of a Parental Attitude Research Instrument." *Child Development,* **29,** 339-361 (1958).
6. Srole, L. "Social Integration and Certain Corollaries: An Exploratory Study". *Amer. Sociol. Rev.,* **21,** 709-716 (1956).
7. *Vital Statistics of the United States, 1963,* Vol. 1: *Natality,* U.S. Department of Health Education and Welfare, Washington, 1964.
8. Lazarus, Richard S. "Cognitive and Personality Factors Underlying Threat and Coping." In *Psychological Stress* Mortimer Appley and Richard Trumbull, eds. Appleton-Century-Crofts, Division of Meredith Publishing Company, New York, 1967, pp. 151-181.

Chapter VI

The Meanings of Motherhood in a Deprived Environment

Eleanor Pavenstedt, M.D.

In order to communicate my impressions of the vicissitudes of motherhood in a poor population, obliged to live in a densely populated, run-down housing project, I must begin by describing the setting of my work during the past year and a half.

This housing project is considered by many of its residents as "the last resort"; it is only too true that families come there who cannot afford to live in private dwellings and who have been turned away from other housing projects.

The 26 high-and low-rise buildings were poorly constructed on made land in Dorchester Bay, part of Boston Harbor. Dump trucks continued to pass through the project, in its early years, to build more land; one of them killed a small child. The mothers thereupon lay down in the street and put an end to this traffic—they anticipated "action" that was to become a key-word in dealing with our poverty population. The recent rat-extermination furor, which led to victory in Congress, was also kindled at Columbia Point. Sudden fury can be unleashed here and is when a woman's children are threatened. (The fact that there are projects now underway to construct middle-and upper-income housing on the same small peninsula impresses one as a real step forward in urban planning.)

The project includes some 1504 units of one to five bedrooms which are customarily occupied. The proximity of the water attracted many old people, who constitute 25% of the population. There are approximately 1128 families with children in the home; over half of these (54%) are female-headed. Some 200 families have children of three and under and approximately 100 infants are born to mothers at Columbia Point each year. There is a turn-over of 14% of the population each year. In the adult segment, whites outnumber Negroes 56 to 44%; among children, however, there are 65% Negroes and 35% whites.

Professors Count Gibson and Jack Geiger of the Tufts Department of Preventive Medicine selected Columbia Point, Massachusetts as the northern urban and Mound Bayou, Mississippi as the southern rural sites for demonstration Health Centers, funded by the Office of Economic Opportunity, in poverty areas. They proposed "to intervene in the cycle of extreme poverty, ill health, unemployment and illiteracy," by providing comprehensive health services. We believe this intervention can be effective only if the health services include mental health in the broadest sense of the word. Our particular interest is in primary prevention, through introducing and fostering child-rearing modalities that will contribute to normal development toward maturity, and thereby help prepare the next generation of adults to assume an active role in their families and in their communities.

The Health Center staff coordinates its services through these Family Health Care groups, each one serving families living in a geographic area assigned to it. The groups consist of a pediatrician, an internist, a social worker, two Public Health nurses, and a non-professional Family Health Aide. As child psychiatrist, I am free to attend any of their daily or more intensive weekly meetings, to which agencies involved with the family under discussion are invited. Through these groups, the Health Center provides an excellent opportunity for becoming acquainted with many of the families. The group meetings also serve to create an important bond with members of the other disciplines, who are eager to share their concerns. The nurses particularly facilitate our making contact with the families. We have made many home visits to test and observe young children and to rate the degree of disorganization in the home, as well as to evaluate the families of older children who were having problems.

THE PROBLEM OF REPEATED PREGNANCIES

As one learns about these families, one particular phenomenon forces itself on one's attention: There are many mothers with myriad problems among their children who seem to have a new child every year. Mrs. W. is a case in point.

> Mrs. W. has nine living children from 12 pregnancies; the eldest, a girl of 23, is removed and has auditory hallucinations. Hospitalization, drugs, and psychotherapy have only succeeded in making her tolerable at home; periodically, she appears at the Health Center because of the voices she hears in her belly. Could these be the voices of the eleven babies she wanted mother to keep in her belly? The next, a 19-year-old boy, grossly retarded, also sits around at home. Another boy, 16, is an emotionally disturbed epileptic, often violent. A 14-year-old girl is very concerned about her small stature, a poor learner, and vicious when teased. An 11-year-old boy is defiant and bullies other children; he too is a poor learner and is so disturbing in class that the school has recommended an institutional placement. The four younger ones, boys of 10 and 9, girls 8 and 4½, are quiet and over-affectionate, in an infantile manner; the 9-and 8-year old have asthma, and one of them has been several times in status asthmaticus and has had pneumonia nine or ten times. The youngest, at 4½, still drinks a bottle at night and sucks her thumb.
>
> Mrs. W. is very concerned that she has not been able to conceive since her husband returned from a TB sanitorium two years ago. She suspects the doctors did something to her at the time of some minor gynecologic repair work. This disorganized woman, whom the nurse describes as affectively removed, managed to diet and lose twenty pounds recently, so that she would be more appealing to her husband, whose interest in sexual relations had abated.
>
> Mrs. W. was raised in an orphanage and by foster par-

> ents. On entering her apartment, one is confronted by a life-size doll on the living room sofa.

When I set out to explore this problem of compulsive pregnancy, and particularly to examine the relationship of these mothers with their infants: whether the pregnancy itself gives them a sense of fulfillment, they are gratified by the early total dependency of the infant, and at what point they disengage themselves and become pregnant again, I soon found that I was treading on very sensitive ground. The poor feel that society denies them the right to have children. No matter what reason the staff put forward to introduce my visit or interview, and regardless of the care I took to weave this inquiry into a lengthy discussion of their problems with their children, they spotted it immediately. One mother, Mrs. P., rebuked me sharply, saying this had nothing to do with the boy's problem about which she had been referred to me. She subsequently broke her son's appointment and allowed some time to elapse before she returned to see her own psychiatrist. A mentally retarded couple were more straight-forward, allowing some discussion of the issue.

> This family has eleven children, five girls placed by Public Welfare and four sons, of whom three are in institutions for the retarded, while the youngest is still at home. Klinefelter's syndrome was identified in several of the boys; recently, the father and two sons were found to have fragile chromosomes. The youngest boy of six, who ran into the room naked during my visit, was spending his mornings in a private special class. Father, resentful about the pediatrician's recommendation to institutionalize him too, said "If I didn't have him, I wouldn't be on welfare."
>
> My visit was motivated by the staff's opinion that every time one of the children was placed, Mrs. D. had had another one. She disabused me by her conscious explanation: "I didn't want them. I couldn't afford them. But my husband used to drink a lot and, when you're drunk, you can't control yourself. So that's how I got them."
>
> On the nurse's next visit she found the D's inquisitive about the reason for my visit. Mrs. D. had figured out

> that I wanted to know whether "she's sexy." Mrs. D. was a thin little wreck of a woman with straggly hair and two teeth.

To attribute multiple conceptions to loss of impulse control alone would most certainly be an oversimplification. Many of the mothers we see complain of frigidity; others feel used by men and hate them for it. Depression and a feeling of isolation drove Mrs. P. repeatedly into the arms of her godfather, a man for whom she had little respect, only to experience intense loneliness and distress following the sexual act. During her pregnancies, depression and feelings of guilt drove her several times to suicidal attempts. Many of the mothers become depressed when they find they are pregnant. Promiscuity with a self-destructive purpose is a frequent outlet for the pent-up emotions of some masochistic, guilt-ridden women (1).

There are others with a certain form of narcissism (1), who feel satisfied only when they are needed, when the children are small and dependent. One told me that, as the children grew older, she felt "put up on the shelf," as she had been in childhood after the arrival of a more beautiful sister.

Another reported, "When I had my first child, I poured everything into my baby. Each time I have a new baby, this happens and I push the older one away." She feels ashamed and humiliated by her marriage to a Negro and says pleadingly that he saved her from prostitution. "He didn't touch me for several months, then approached me gently." Like all the other couples of mixed marriages that I have become acquainted with here, the X's engage in violent fighting. Stirred to anger, she lashes out with easily available insults and invectives that fall on sensitized ears and rouse her Negro husband to a blind fury. The mother then turns to her babies for emotional release; but as soon as they are old enough to be outside and seen by neighbors, Mrs. X's feelings from the other side of her ambivalence become apparent in her projections. She keeps her children close, isolates them from playmates, and limits their range of activities. Eventually they get in each other's hair, at such close quarters, and her screaming and blows burst forth indiscriminately. It has been written that the poor seldom verbalize their feelings. The intensity of this woman's emotions came across with tremendous impact during our initial interview. This intensity was further illustrated by her reaction to the news that a 13-year-old boy had been drowned off the project: she packed her six children into a car and drove all the way to New York with them, arriving back home at 3 A.M.

THE FEELING OF THE RIGHT OF POOR MOTHERS TO KEEP THEIR CHILDREN

In this past year and a half, I have begun to reconsider my previous attitude about forcibly removing neglected children from their mothers. Practically, our experience with placement agencies at Columbia Point, seems to show that they cannot meet the demand—perhaps because they were not prepared for the population explosion, or because, with our recent attention to the poor, we are entering many homes previously passed by unnoticed, homes where children are exposed to destructive influences. Our first impulse was to remove them, but this proved to be impossible in most instances.

It seems as though personnel responsible for taking children from "unfit homes" experience guilty feelings, for they usually placed only grossly neglected babies, girls in puberty who were in sexual danger, and boys who had already committed delinquent acts—and, without much reason, left behind others who were destined for the same fate, but might still have been modifiable.

There are some mothers who end by almost begging us to place their children—for example, boys around ten (there was even a six year old), whom the schools have excluded, who defy their mother's control, and who have frequent encounters with the police. We also had one mother who, out of her own pathological conflicts, placed an infant son for adoption. For each one of these, there are ten others who avoid contact with anyone who may want to "take my children away," and fight, through every channel open to them, to have the children returned. No matter how negligent, how devoid of contact or communication with them, how abusive they may be, these mothers cling to their children.

In response to the questions: what do these children represent to their mothers, why do they defend their right to keep them with such ferocity, many people say, "These women are so deprived, they have nothing else." Surely this is part of the answer, but the women must have other motives than the need for possessions. Previously we had thought that ill-defined limits between the self and the child made every separation into a painful mutilation, but this is difficult to establish.

The statement of a mentally retarded, alcoholic, promiscuous, and sometimes violent mother of nine children has stayed with me. Periodically, Mrs. C. would become so agitated and distraught that she would demand to have her children placed while she sought admission to a state hospital for herself. Once she came home before the children had been returned. "I didn't know what to do with myself. I sat there smoking, feeling helpless and useless. Without the children, I had no life." In other words, her children are her only link to reality or perhaps even constitute her reality. They fill her life with activity, no matter how disorganized; their empty stomachs punctuate her day. Without them, she is faced with emptiness and passivity; her self-disparagement becomes unremitting.

Usually the mother's distress and resentment is shared by her children, who are also filled with anxiety over what awaits them. Even though many a deprived mother withdraws from her children when they no longer fulfill her needs, early bonds are not completely dissolved. A threat from outside the home can revive them, since in a way such a threat makes the children again dependent on her powers of protection.

In the home of one mother, wanted in another state for attempting to stab a man, the children are openly hostile to visitors from the Health Center, laughing at them, making deprecating comments, and even hitting and poking at them.

This mother is deathly afraid that her children will be taken from her. Yet, when we went to the back bedroom to see her baby and he lifted his arms to be picked up, she said to me "He always do that" and explained that she avoided picking him up lest he annoy her with his crying. There wasn't a toy in the house. Does this mother need her children to confirm her hostility, to share it with her so that she be not completely isolated?

BACKGROUND FINDINGS IN CHRONIC PROBLEM FAMILIES

Mental retardation is present in the largest group of families that give us constant concern. Psychosis of a parent or the mental breakdown of a grandparent during the parent's childhood is the next most frequent finding. Another recurrent event is the history of orphanage or foster-home placement of the mother early in life. It is precisely this finding that has led me to question our reliance on placement away from home as a treatment measure. Most of the mothers who were placed during their childhood are extremely fragile; they have little energy to cope with their family or are chronically depressed or both.

We will, of course, never be able entirely to eliminate placement of children away from home. I have come to doubt the benefit of it, especially for children from poor, deprived families. Both parents and children experience it as being dispossessed of their rights by an authoritarian society. They see their mothers totally shorn of power to protect them, and their feelings of powerlessness and worthlessness are intensified. For those who again encounter rejection from foster parents, sometimes repeatedly, the experience is devastating.

PROGRAMS THAT COMPLEMENT HOME CARE

Our task at this time is, I believe, to establish programs that will complement child-rearing in the home. At Columbia

Point, we are planning a Day Care Unit for infants and toddlers. The infant unit will be supervised by a nurse with maternal and child health training, and the toddler unit by a graduate of an early childhood education program. The need for the infant unit became clear as the staff attempted to support psychotic and otherwise seriously disturbed mothers of infants. But beyond this group, children in the second and third year of life, by and large, receive a minimum of understanding, stimulation, and training at Columbia Point. The development of autonomy, which depends on some recognition by the environment of a child's need to manage himself and his affairs, with assistance from adults, is completely thwarted. Even if the importance of curiosity and exploration were recognized, overcrowding would permit very little of it. Routine, order, and consistency are lacking in many of the homes. Speech development and the habit of communicating can also be fostered at the unit.

Space does not permit our having a center for the whole family, but whenever there are children absent we will encourage other family members to come. There will be small rooms with one-way mirrors for viewing each age-group. Mothers will be invited to watch their children from these, and a staff member will be present to respond to their comments and attempt gradually to gain their acceptance of our handling of the children. There will be a training unit for one of the "new professions." Mature women from poverty areas will receive a year of training in healthy child-rearing, child care, and the elements of nursing and child psychology. They will accompany staff members who go into the children's homes to help the mothers deal with their children in ways that will further their development. Together they will explore how much of the practices carried out with the children in the unit are compatible with the life of the family. We expect that, following their graduation, these Family Change Agents will work in housing projects and slum areas, assisting social workers, nurses, and pediatricians by working with mothers and children in the homes of families that arouse concern. As we make contact with more and more families, we plan to have many discussion groups. Our Health

Action staff has talked about developing a local closed-circuit TV channel, and we plan to work on some child-rearing programs.

Before ending, I would like to discuss some possibilities for coping with our present impasse in the management of deprived children.

Several states have established *departments* for the welfare of children. In these, public support of the deprived, care of the handicapped and neglected, and programing for delinquent children are under one roof. There are many children from slum areas involved in minor delinquent activities, whom our courts are reluctant to adjudicate as delinquents and who would actually not profit from our present institutions. Many of them are not really neglected—the parents (often mothers alone) simply can't control them without help. Furthermore, law enforcement agencies are so concerned with adolescent gangs that little is done to work preventively with young children who stray away from home, ride all day on public conveyances, climb into dangerous places, and commit minor acts of vandalism.

Marguerite Q. Warren's Community Treatment Project for delinquent youths would, I believe, be equally suitable for the so-called neglected and for younger children. She and her staff have classified juvenile offenders according to their "interpersonal maturity level." They have worked out a differential plan of treatment and described the personal characteristics needed to treat children belonging to nine subtypes. They work with many modalities: day care, foster homes, and small group homes, avoiding large institutions and returning the subjects to their own homes as soon as possible. Their rate of recidivism is lower for all but one subtype as compared with a control group from institutions.

If all children requiring public intervention were dealt with by one agency, it might well attract sophisticated and inspired leadership. The operations of the entire department could then be developed from a theoretical developmental scheme similar to or the same as the one described above which is being used in California.

REFERENCE

1. Deutsch, Helene, *Psychology of Women*, Vol. 11. Grune & Stratton, New York, 1915, Chapter X.

Section 3

Programs to Assist Parents

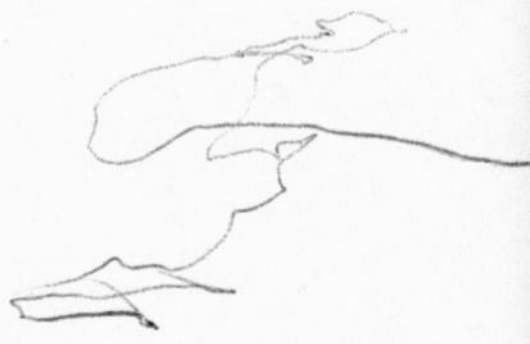

Introduction

Previous chapters have made recommendations for change and called for programs. This section includes two papers outlining original and creative efforts to improve the plight of seriously deprived families and their children.

The first comes from the Philadelphia Child Guidance Clinic; its author, Charles A. Malone, M.D., is Training Director as well as Associate Professor of Clinical Child Psychiatry at the University of Pennsylvania Medical School. I shall let Dr. Malone speak for himself: "This paper will describe and discuss the services being conducted by the Philadelphia Child Guidance Clinic in the urban slum in which it is located. Beginning with a presentation of demographic data that will outline the 'face of poverty' in South Philadelphia, the paper will characterize certain of the gross mental health problems noted in this slum area, particularly those related to serious family disorganization. The heart of the paper will focus on the child psychiatric service innovations that the Clinic is developing to meet these problems: cognitive skill training for underachieving children; group therapy for illegitimately pregnant young adolescent school dropouts; in-service training of elementary school teachers concerning the impediments to learning that occur in slum families; sensitization of pediatricians to the dimensions of family disorganization and their impact on health and child-rearing practices; and the development of indigenous neighborhood aides who provide leadership in local self-help mobilization and organization.

"In discussing several innovations in greater detail, emphasis will be placed on elucidating, where possible, the principles that underlie these innovations, how they are based on an understanding of disorganized, low socioeconomic family life, and how they modify the staff's view of child psychiatry."

The final chapter describes what can be done, even in a huge city like New York, when an executive has the know-how to gain the support of sufficiently influential and dedicated people; when she has a clear well-organized thought process, so that the problem is set clearly before them; and when all of them have the energy to bring into being a creative practical program to at least cushion the trauma of separation for children and speed up assistance to them.

The work of the Community Council of Greater New York deserves respect for what it has called attention to and for its success in taking action where a kind of hopeless lethargy had hitherto prevailed.

Chapter VII

Child Psychiatric Services in an Urban Slum

Charles A. Malone, M.D.

Developing effective services in an urban slum is one of the most significant and urgent tasks confronting child psychiatry today. Across the nation, broad community mental health programs are being instituted, planned, or contemplated. In view of the distressing fact that one of the ugly features of the face of poverty in any city is the vicious generation-after-generation cycle of severe psychosocial pathology, a vital part of many of these programs is, or will be, aimed at relieving or removing the complex, chronic mental health problems that abound in slums. The need for and importance of these efforts is unquestionable, yet their outcome is clearly in doubt. This is largely because the serious nature of the mental health problems that must be met in developing effective services challenges our knowledge and professional competence to their limits. It is also because the development of useful services in a slum area must be an integral part of broader efforts to ameliorate the effects of poverty, and this requirement challenges our capacity as a society to its limits.

Beyond the enormous difficulty involved in meeting the complex mental health problems in a slum, work in this area is impeded by certain features of the atmosphere that surrounds community psychiatry. We are all familiar with these features, which are present (to a greater or lesser extent) in different urban communities: There is an urgency nowadays to set up community mental health services that are *completely* new and different—a need to conceive of them as unconnected with the past and "untainted" by tradition; there are frantic efforts to get into the community psychiatry business in a big way (this often leads to irresponsible vested interest arguments over who is going to be "responsible" for which 200,000 population "catchment" area); at times, there are service experimentations that appear based on a disillusionment with treatment; and there is a tendency to interpret *comprehensive* services not only as "large in scope," but as meeting all the mental health needs of large populations, regardless of age, type of pathology, level of family organization, and socioeconomic status.

These trends often lead to an unnecessary and unproductive dichotomy between the past and the present, between traditional concepts and techniques and service innovations. One result of this is that familiar mental health problems are *referred* for traditional services, and this further overburdens an already overworked referral system and adds to unmanageable waiting lists. These trends also frequently stir up polemic disputes and territorial rivalries in mental health service areas that require the most mature and thoughtful cooperation, coordination, and integration. This tendency appears likely to produce a bureaucratic overlay of still another layer of fragmented, diffuse, "too little and too late" services. These misdirections regarding community mental health services have been mentioned because psychiatric programs in urban areas must contend with them and must manage to avoid their impeding effects.

The purpose of this paper is to share the ongoing experience of the Philadelphia Child Guidance Clinic (1) in developing services in the slum neighborhood in which it is located. We shall present aspects of the community mental health work in which we are engaged in order to illustrate certain problems and issues that have emerged and to communicate some of the viewpoints and premises that underlie this work. It is our belief that the challenge and complexity of this kind of work requires the pooling and evaluation of clinical experience from various programs in different urban slums. In view of the desperate need for this service, there is a strong temptation in this area to *act first and think later*. Consequently we believe that it is important to intensify our efforts to distill from our ongoing experience meaningful generalizations that can be thoughtfully evaluated, challenged, and modified.

Our Clinic is located in the midst of a Negro ghetto in one of Philadelphia's worst slum areas. A few demographic data will outline several of the gross features of the face of poverty in our community:

One-half the families have an income below $3,000 per year; one-third of the families are on public assistance, and many of these are *hard-core* families and second-or third-generation families on welfare; nearly 50% of the housing is seriously substandard; the average schooling level is eighth grade; half the households are without an adult male.

In an effort to ameliorate the untoward effects of poverty on families in our neighborhood, the Clinic has placed increasing emphasis on developing community service programs over the last two years. The need for such services is enormous, as witnessed by the kinds of incidence of severe psychosocial pathology that occur in the area surrounding the Clinic:

Of the births, 40% are illegitimate; only one-fourth of the homes are stable; delinquency, crime, and venereal disease rates are among the highest in the city; there is also a high incidence of mental hospitalization, alcoholism, and drug addiction.

The Clinic has attempted to respond to this pressing need for help by reserving one-half of its service for low-income families from the neighborhood. This has involved us in continuing efforts to use a variety and combination of investigative, therapeutic, and educational modalities to provide increasingly effective service to poor families. It has also provided us with a background of clinical skills that serve as a foundation for the new programs we are developing in our neighborhood.

Over the past two years we have established a number of services: a family health clinic; consultation to poverty-program nursery schools; group therapy for illegitimately pregnant school dropouts; cognitive skills training for underachieving children; parent education groups; a program for the development of indigenous neighborhood aides; in-service training for elementary school teachers; aftercare for children discharged from residential treatment; and naturalistic studies of family life and social "networks" of families in the neighborhood. While some of these services cover the entire section of South Philadelphia which the Clinic serves, most of them are concentrated in the same public school district that is a smaller geographical area adjacent to the Clinic.

In order to describe this community service meaningfully, certain premises and views that we hold regarding it must be made explicit: The gross statistics regarding the incidence of mental illness underscore the fact that there are so many complex and serious problems in the area we serve that, no matter how extensive our program becomes, it cannot expect to meet the mental health needs of our neighborhood. Consequently, we have chosen to establish small, manageable, carefully demarcated programs, which enable us to concentrate our efforts. This avoids overwhelming size and complexity which overburden and discourage staff. In view of the sizable discrepancy between the supply of clinic manpower and the demand for service, we often set up each service program as a pilot study, in which large problem areas are met on a smaller scale.

Gradually a small program, if it is effective, spreads to touch upon other related and contiguous mental health problem areas. These new areas can be included in the community service program of the clinic, wherever the clinic and community resources are adequate. Where clinic and neighborhood resources are inadequate to provide needed services in these new areas, however, a valuable feedback indicating the need for new facilities can be given to the community.

In relation to this latter point, it seems to us important to clarify for the community we serve what we *cannot* do—including the limitations of our knowledge and skill—as well as what we can do. We must be careful not to stimulate interest in services that cannot be provided or sustained. In this regard, it seems necessary to avoid using the already overburdened referral system wherever possible. We must avoid being drawn into a process of "picking up the pieces" and doing our best in relation to mental health problems where the prospect of repair or even salvage is virtually nil. Where the child and family health care provisions and resources of a community are woefully inadequate, problems develop faster than they can be treated. Responsible governmental and private funding agencies must be informed about these situations and must take them into account since, under these circumstances, child psychiatric services, no matter how well conceived, are destined to be too little and too late.

It has seemed important for our neighborhood services to develop out of the interest and skills of the staff, rather than be superimposed and "forced," in order simply to accommodate to the availability of federal or state funds. The addition to our staff of disciplines beyond those of the traditional child guidance team has been invaluable in broadening the foundation of staff skills needed in developing our services. A remedial teacher has been instrumental in planning and conducting our work with "slow learners"; a community organization worker has been vital in developing local citizen participation and support for our work; a marriage counsellor-educator has been involved in our parent education groups; an anthropologist has been responsible for our family studies.

No matter how many additions we make to our staff, however, the gap between available child psychiatric manpower and the need for mental health services will remain large. Consequently, we need to discover in our community program effective means of collaboration and training that will extend the competence of non-mental health professionals in dealing with the emotional aspects of childhood and family problems they come in contact with in their daily work.

SERVICES IN THE SLUM COMMUNITY

Having presented this background of the atmosphere regarding community psychiatry in which we work and the views and premises that underlie our services, we shall now describe and discuss several community programs that the Clinic is conducting. These services illustrate several issues and problems with which we have been confronted in the difficult process of developing child psychiatric services in a slum neighborhood.

1. Cognitive Skills Training for Underachieving Children *

In an elementary school near the Clinic, we have been conducting and comparing the effectiveness of different approaches to groups of fourth- and fifth-graders whose basic skills and achievement levels are two to three-and-a-half years behind the national average for their grade. All the children in the program are Negro, and slightly over half are boys. One group of twelve children, found to be hyperactive in an initial psychiatric and neurological screening of both grades, are receiving Dexidrene (2). Three groups of eight children each come to the Clinic once a week for modified group psychotherapy. These group sessions are aimed at increasing the youngsters' trust in relations with grownups and their ability to observe themselves and others, as well as what is happening around them. The sessions are particularly focused on relationships and on a developing awareness of the impact of feelings on themselves and each other. We aim particularly at eliciting painful feelings that may have a bearing on school performance—for instance, profound feelings of devaluation, inadequacy, and incompetence, or feelings of anger related to frustration, or "scared" feelings related to the dangers of the neighborhood. Three other groups of eight children each come to the Clinic once a week for group sessions run by a remedial teacher. These sessions aim at teaching the youngsters specific cognitive skills within an enjoyable "game" format. Finally, there are two groups of eight children each who have the

* This program is an adaptation of techniques developed by Minuchin *et al.* (3). It was introduced in the Clinic by Pamela Chamberlain and carried on by members of our staff: T. Pierce, A. Barcal, and E. Hirsh.

same amount of time as the other groups but spend it in an enjoyable art class with an interested and responsive teacher. These latter two groups are intended to serve as controls in the process of comparing the overall effectiveness of each type of group. *

Let us describe in greater detail the groups aimed at teaching cognitive skills (3). These groups are aimed at improving the children's basic skills, stimulating their interest in and enjoyment from learning, increasing their capacity to adjust their behavior to "classroom" expectations, and providing them with opportunities to experience themselves as competent in some aspects of problem-solving. These goals are based on our understanding of the youngsters' characteristic functioning in school. These Negro children exhibit the impediments to effective learning found among low socioeconomic children that have been described in the literature (4-7): limited attention, inadequate concentration, and short memory span; limited language skills; global, poorly differentiated communication, which is oriented to affect, relationship, and status rather than content; concrete action-oriented thinking; poor capacity for self-observation and judgment; and a tendency to restless, provocative behavior. Using a game format, the teacher emphasizes use of the senses, listening, asking questions, remembering sequences, communicating in words, and task completion (3). In this process, interest, effort, and partial success in the direction of the group goal are identified and credited by the teacher. The teacher communicates that she "means business" by her serious interest in learning and tries to avoid controlling, authoritarian positions. When the children reveal increasing mastery, the teacher gradually introduces more formal learning tasks resembling their school work, until they are actually undertaking problems that are at or near their grade level.

Another aspect of this project involves efforts to assist the children to improve their capacity to observe themselves and

* The results of this comparison are being prepared for separate publication.

others and to use judgment. We work toward this by having two of the eight children go behind the one-way mirror with a staff member, in order to rate the remaining six children in their functioning. The ratings are of performance in the use of cognitive skills and behavior in the "classroom," with the emphasis on performance. The two judges and the staff member independently rate the children on their performance (including interest, effort, and partial success) in accomplishing the different aspects of the goal involved in the game or schoolwork tasks. The staff member compares his ratings with those of the judges and assists them in articulating the basis for their judgment. The judges can make changes in their ratings on the basis of this comparison, if they wish. The ratings are then shared with the other youngsters. By rotating the task of judging, all the children gain experience and develop skills in observing and judging and in communicating the results in words. Through this judging process, the children's judgment regarding achievement may become emancipated from its ties to the parent-child interaction with which they are familiar in their homes and become appropriately connected to problem-solving activities. With regard to the rating of "classroom" behavior, we attempt to move the children from their usual position or preoccupation with "bad" versus "good" behavior to observing whether behavior interferes with adequate performance or facilitates it.

This group approach to improving cognitive skills in underachieving, low socioeconomic Negro fourth-and fifth-graders, as part of a larger study, was initiated with built-in means for data collection and analysis to evaluate its effectiveness. Despite the difficulties involved in evaluation and the cost in staff time in carrying it out, we are convinced that this is necessary in neighborhood services to slum children. The pressing need of the population served and the amount of self-investment the services require may lead to self-deceptive impressions of significant changes in the children. Clinical impressions of improvement or the lack of it must be supported by objective data. False optimism or discouragement can lead us astray. For example, although the data analysis is incomplete, it appears that our clinical optimism about the modified group psychotherapy approach will not be as well supported by objective data as will our optimism about the groups aimed at improving cognitive skills. The objective confirmation of our clinical impression of significant gains in the latter approach strengthens our confidence in deciding to increase the staff-time commitment to this type of service.

This type of child psychiatric service to underachieving local school children has a number of advantages. To begin with, it is proving to be a means of providing a substantial degree of effective help to four children, utilizing one hour per week of staff-time for approximately six months. It may serve as a model for the training of teachers. The professional skills and techniques involved in this type of service appear to be ones that can be taught to a group of public school teachers. It seems likely that we shall explore this possibility, generally or selectively, in our in-service training program for elementary school teachers (described below). It certainly is a model for staff training. Several staff members have already learned the techniques and are able to employ them with groups of underachievers. It has made the whole staff more keenly aware of the possibilities of stimulating learning skills and the importance of actual experiences of intellectual competence in their work with underachieving slum children.

2. Family Health Clinic *

In cooperation with Children's Hospital, we have established a clinic to provide medical and mental health care for seven hundred slum families, many of whom are unable to make effective use of existing medical facilities. The clinic utilizes indigenous neighborhood aides who live and work in the community to reach out to disorganized families needing health

* This program is part of the Rebound Children and Youth Services Project, under the direction of P. Wilson, with L. Wechsler as mental health coordinator.

care and to serve as a liaison between such families and the clinic. Using shared clinical experience, which demonstrates characteristics of low socioeconomic family life, this program aims at sensitizing pediatricians to the dimensions of family maladaptation and disorganization and their impact on health and child-rearing practices. Through this type of conjoint work with child psychiatrists, the skills of pediatricians in working with such families are gradually extended.

The family health clinic plays an important role in gaining community support for our child psychiatric services. Experience seems to be proving that grass-roots interest and support is essential for services in a slum to be effective. Developing community involvement in a population that is dispossessed and alienated, however, is particularly difficult: There is an atmosphere of distrust, suspicion, hopelessness, and defeat; low levels of individual family and group initiative and assertion, combined with apathy and a sense of powerlessness, delay the process of neighborhood organization. Developing community support for services is all the more difficult because there is a history of service gaps that have ignored the needs of the poor; services have frequently been organized with a middle-class bias, so that receiving help has involved devaluing experiences for low-income families. Promoting community involvement in service programs is further complicated by the fact that those who step forward and claim to represent the poor are often political opportunists seeking their own ends or militant leaders, who, with some justification, oppose the service as a middle-class means of maintaining the status quo.

The family health clinic has been at the hub of our attempts to cope with these impediments to community support. Among the possible avenues of service to the population in our neighborhood, we chose to emphasize the areas of health and education, partly because previous experience had led us to the conclusion that these were areas in which distrust and suspicion were lowest and hopes highest. Health services are direct, concrete, and relieving; they are available twenty-four hours a day. Families are likely to have had previous experience receiving medical help that did not require or ask for an "acceptable" pedigree.

From the outset, representatives of the community have participated in the planning of the family health clinic program. This has engaged us in the at times difficult process of achieving a working cooperation with the organized elements of the community, while avoiding the attempts of political opportunists to gain control.

A central part of the family health clinic services involves the selection and in-service training of people who live in the area to work as *neighborhood aides*. A major focus of the work of these aides is to assist in the development of block organizations and neighborhood leaders. Initially aimed at promoting communication and social activity, these block organizations became increasingly geared to self-help and action to change local conditions. This type of organization can be a stimulus for local group efforts to effect their environment, including the nature of the services available in our program. This may lead to criticism or attacks on our program. It remains to be seen whether or not we will have the maturity to understand and respond to these trial-and-error efforts of the poor to have an influential voice in the planning and conduct of health services, if and when they come.

3. In-Service Training for Elementary School Teachers *

In collaboration with the Philadelphia Public School System, we are conducting a voluntary in-service training program for eighteen of the twenty teachers working in a nearby elementary school. The school, which has a 100% Negro population, has been designated by the Board of Education as one of the most depressed and needy schools in the city. Our program was designed primarily to sensitize the teachers to the developmental characteristics and the patterns of family life of the low socioeconomic children in their classrooms which have a bearing on the youngsters' ability to learn and adjust

* This work is conducted by S. Minuchin, B. Montalvo, P. Minuchin, and N. Daniels.

in school. In small groups with a staff member, the teachers observe a series of four or five consecutive semi-structured interviews involving volunteer low socioeconomic families with one or more children having learning problems at school. In the different semi-structured interviews, we attempt to demonstrate as best we can such things as: patterns of relationship and communication in the family; attitudes toward learning; how the family approaches and deals with tasks requiring joint solution; the children's cognitive skills; and how mothers go about teaching their children how to solve a problem. These observations form a basis of shared experiences for group discussion between the teachers and clinic staff. The teachers learn to distinguish similarities and differences between the children's home and school environments. The teachers are surprised, for instance, when they realize that they are often unwittingly drawn into dealing with the children in the same controlling, authoritative and, at times, punitive manner as the parents do. Thus they recognize that they have been perpetuating certain family patterns that can interfere with learning.

It is interesting to observe the development of a meaningful group process among the teachers. Previously, they had not been in the habit of exchanging their ideas concerning teaching. This had led to a virtual "coalition of ignorance," in which misconceptions, misinformation, and ineffectual teaching techniques persisted through silence and circumspection. As the process of discussing the observations and comparing teaching experiences begins to take hold, this coalition of ignorance gives way. The teachers begin to acknowledge their need to learn, to share common problems, and to offer useful suggestions regarding successful or unsuccessful techniques. The teachers have a tendency to resist their own active involvement in learning, by treating the training as though it were a didactic course and appealing to us as the "experts" to tell them what to do. Although it is difficult for them, they are responsive when they begin to turn to themselves and each other as resources in meeting educational problems and to discover that they have more actual or potential competence than they had previously recognized.

In relation to our goal of sensitizing the teachers to the learning handicaps of the children, a major obstacle involves devaluing attitudes and bias against lower-class Negroes, which exist among a number of the teachers. This was particularly noticeable among several middle-class Negro teachers (about half of the total group of teachers are Negro). They seem to need to distinguish themselves from "bad" Negroes and to react against their own earlier lower-class background. For example, a Negro mother favorably evaluated by the teachers in various aspects of her parental functioning with her youngster was generally condemned in relation to her child-care practices when the group learned that she had been promiscuous. Several of the Negro teachers put forward the thesis that the most important thing they could teach the children was to be polite and well-behaved. Developing intellectual resources for effective problem-solving ranked well below being quiet and "good" in the educational values of these teachers. In view of the bias that existed in some of the teachers, one can imagine how stormy, painful, and discouraging some of the group discussions were. Despite the strain and difficulty this produced, however, it was invaluable in demonstrating some of the mismatch and antagonism that exists for the children in relation to the differences between their home and school environments. It also demonstrated the perpetuation of family patterns that overemphasize control and "good" versus "bad" behavior, as well as the children's own tendency to evaluate behavior in these terms. Struggling with the teachers' attitudes made us particularly aware of the importance of teacher participation in the planning of their own in-service training (something that we hadn't given sufficient emphasis to in our original format for the program). On the basis of their evaluation of the pros and cons of the program, the teachers and the clinic staff are jointly planning the next phase of their in-service training.

The in-service training of teachers has yielded an unexpected feedback, which may affect the Clinic's approach to low socioeconomic families. We mentioned earlier that parents who had one or more children underachieving at school volunteered to participate in this program to help teachers understand the needs of underachieving children better. These parents did not consider themselves patients and we noted that they were less problem-oriented and defensive in presenting themselves than parents usually are when they come to the Clinic. We also noted that the staff members who interviewed them were also less pathology-oriented and were more geared to the families' assets and potentials. There seemed to be more respect for the parents' capacity to be active in helping their children. Almost all these parents requested an opportunity to continue to come to the Clinic to receive this type of "help."

This raises interesting questions: Could we work more effectively with certain low-income families if they and we did not view them as "patients"? Do we inadvertantly slip into a "set" of "you are the patient— I am the active healer" that interferes with our clinical work, especially with lower-class families who are not socially adapted to being clinic patients? Certainly low-income families appear to be extra-sensitive to devaluation and to being helpless. Being a volunteer may prove to be a more comfortable basis on which such families can come to the Clinic. In any event, we need to explore working with families and children who are "not patients" in order to learn more about these phenomena.

4. Group Therapy for Unwed Young Adolescent Mothers *

Any program of child psychiatric services in an urban slum must take into account the crucial issue of community need; it must respond to local need and offer services in relation to problems that the community defines as serious and urgent. One such problem in our community involves adolescent girls who have illegitimate children. During their pregnancy, these girls are forced to leave school. Usually coming from unstable, disorganized homes, they wander aimlessly about the

* This program is conducted by P. Miranda and J. Morrow.

neighborhood, lacking a place to go or something to do. They are unwanted girls carrying unwanted babies. Before they have accomplished the developmental tasks of childhood, let alone successfully engaged in the issues of adolescence, these young girls must become mothers. To add to their enormous psychological troubles, they often lack models of adequate mothering in their own experience. Instead, their lives have yielded other models—ones in which bits of tenderness, affection, and loving care are confusingly mixed with inconstancy, unreliability, impulsivity, and hostility. The lack of differentiation between the generations and the generation-after-generation repetition of certain forms of pathology that is frequently found in their families confronts us with a powerful vicious cycle.

Our service in relation to this difficult and sizable problem area is limited. On a pilot study basis, we are offering group therapy to eight young adolescent unwed mothers. The group therapy is conducted by a pediatrician and by one of our staff members who is experienced in group therapy. Some of the sessions involve only the young adolescents; in other sessions, they bring their babies. Some sessions involve mainly verbal exchange among the group pertaining to individual and interpersonal problems that the girls have in common; other sessions center around direct demonstrations of infant care. The brief flashes of maternal concern and tenderness, of briefly restored self-esteem, of the girls' confused struggle to find themselves that emerge in the sessions are poignant and deeply touching.

Among the interesting things illustrated by this service is the reciprocal benefit that this type of mental health professional-pediatrician collaboration demonstrates. Too frequently, in the past, the cooperation between child psychiatry and pediatrics has been impeded by territorialism and rivalry. Even when cooperation in common problem areas does occur, the labor is divided rather strictly along discipline-prerogative lines. Too frequently we work in parallel with each other, rather than conjointly. As much as the traditional division of labor makes obvious sense, it limits the expansion of horizons in each discipline. Mental health professionals and pediatricians will not learn what they need to learn from each other and modify their professional resources as they need to modify them, if they continue to limit their collaboration to reports, case conferences, and consultation, and their reciprocal training to lectures and seminars. Child psychiatric personnel and pediatric personnel need to have opportunities to work side by side.

In this service, where the group therapy is being conducted conjointly, reciprocal avenues of professional exchange are necessary and required. The pediatrician is learning about group processes and dynamics. She is learning techniques for promoting interaction, exploring the dimensions of emotional problems, and intervening to produce desired effects. The pediatrician is also discovering that her own expertise goes well beyond her knowledge of medicine. She is realizing that her knowledge about child care can become a means of helping these adolescent girls emotionally, as well as practically. She is recognizing that her natural womanly response to the girls and their difficulties can be an effective psychological technique. Our staff member is also learning. He is discovering that the expertise of the pediatrician is not mysterious and need not be obscure to anyone without a medical degree; he is learning that her freedom to deal directly with physical care is useful from a psychological point of view; he is realizing that some of her simple, human responses are therapeutic, and that his expertise in group therapy does not preclude his learning techniques from her. This model of side-by-side conjoint work appears to hold far greater potential for realizing the goals of collaboration between pediatrics and child psychiatry than the previous models we have used.

SUMMARY

The experience of the Philadelphia Child Guidance Clinic in conducting child psychiatric services in the urban slum in which it is located has been described as a means of illustrating some of the general and local problems that emerge in this type of complex and difficult work. Current trends and attitudes about community mental health that lead to unnecessary dichotomies, irresponsible rivalries, and unproductive disputes were mentioned. Emphasis was placed on the premises and viewpoints on which the community services are based—that manageable, carefully demarcated pilot programs, which concentrate staff efforts and can be studied, are preferred; that it is important for services to grow out of staff interest and skills, and to determine what we cannot do, as well as what we can do; that programs need to aim at increasing the competence of non-mental health personnel in dealing with mental health problems; and that the very nature and complexity of the service goals require that we evaluate the effectiveness of programs.

Four areas of service in a slum neighborhood—cognitive skills training for underachievers; a family health clinic; in-service training for teachers; and group therapy for unwed young adolescent mothers—were described briefly to illustrate issues that have emerged. In describing the general issues underscored by the Clinic's experience with these services, stress has been laid on the difficulties involved in developing community support; the importance of basing clinical work on an understanding of the psychosocial characteristics of the low socioeconomic population served; the impediment of bias against lower-class Negroes; the necessity of objective confirmation or refutation of clinical impressions; and the value of conjoint work with pediatricians.

REFERENCES

1. Malone, C. A. "Child Psychiatric Services for Low Socioeconomic Families." *J. Amer. Acad. Child Psychiat,* **6,** No. 2, 332-345 (1967).
2. Conners, C. K., Eisenberg, L., and Barcai, A. "Effect of Dextroamphetamine on Children: Studies on Subjects with Learning Disabilities and School Behavior Problems." *Arch. Gen. Psychiatry,* **17,** 478-486 (1961).
3. Minuchin, S., Chamberlain, P., and Graubard, P. "A Project to Teach Learning Skills to Disturbed, Delinquent Children." *Amer. J. Orthopsychiatry,* **37,** No. 3, 558-567 (1967).

4. Bernstein, B., "Social Class and Linguistic Development: A Theory of Social Learning." In: *Education, Economy and Society* (A. H. Halsey, Jr. Floud and C. A. Anderson, eds.) Free Press, New York, 1963, pp. 288-314.
5. Hess, R. D., and Shipman, V. C. "Early Experience and the Socialization of Cognitive Modes in Children." *Child Development,* **36,** 869-886 (1965).
6. Malone, C. A., Pavenstedt, E., Mattick, I., Bandler, L., Stein, M. and Mintz, N. *The Drifters: Children of Lower Class Families.* Little, Brown and Co., Boston, 1967.
7. Minuchin, S. "Psychoanalytic Therapies and the Low Socioeconomic Population." In *Modern Psychoanalysis: New Directions and Perspectives* J. Marmor, ed. Basic Books, New York, 1968.

Chapter VIII

Parental Incapacity and the Welfare of Children

A Report on a Community Effort to Stem the Tide of Children Going Into Foster Care

Roberta Hunt, M.S.W.

I am impressed with the degree to which psychiatrists and welfare workers are battling in a common cause and, though starting from different points, coming to similar conclusions. The study and the subsequent follow-up activity that I want to report grows out of a commitment to the welfare of children, and particularly to securing for them the values and the protections of good parental care when—for whatever reason—their own parents, without help, cannot meet their needs. But, you will say, what I have just described is a mental-health-program objective. I would certainly agree. Psychiatry and social work *do* clearly share a common conviction about the importance of the early years. We would agree I am sure that the quality of experience in early childhood, particularly the child's experience with parental care, is a crucial determinant of his later social functioning. It is a crucial variant in forecasting potential for mental health or for mental illness; in forecasting a potential for good parenthood, or in predicting parental failure or incapacity. Wherever our individual point of entry as professionals, in terms of our primary interest or concern, we come upon a circle that leads—to or from—the continuity and quality of parental care.

What a community decides to do, therefore, to protect children from abuse, or from the less dramatic but in the long run equally serious and far more extensive problems of neglect or grossly inadequate care, will have a direct effect on what that community may eventually expect to harvest. The neglected or mistreated child will reappear with disturbing frequency in the caseload of disturbed and neglectful parents. Yesterday's poorly resolved child-care and protection problems are already on our doorsteps today.

The study * on which I am directing a follow-up "action" project was not prompted primarily by concern over the growing numbers of mentally ill, neglectful, or abusive parents, although it did document vivid and appalling evidence of the prevalence and repetivences of these problems in New York City. This study was prompted by desperation over the chronically overcrowded conditions at the shelters the community maintains to receive children caught in child-care crisis situations of all kinds. And there was concern also about the chronic inability of social service agencies—either governmental or voluntary—to begin to fully meet needs for help to families when, for whatever reason, there is a breakdown in parental capacity.

The major thrust of the study was to prevent foster-care placement. The gap between foster care needs and foster care resources in New York City has been labeled a national scandal and a disgrace. The hand-wringing and haranguing about it—as well as the heroic efforts to stretch, expand, and strengthen foster care resources—had gone on for so long without significant results that the very chronicity of the problem made it harder to resolve. The problem had been "studied to death," too, but the focus had usually been on possibilities for expansion of foster care resources, or as our electronics-minded colleagues would say, on foster care "outputs" rather than "inputs."

---

* A report on the *Paths to Child Placement* study, by Dr. Shirley Jenkins and Mignon Sauber, was published in 1966 by the Community Council of Greater New York. The study was co-sponsored by the Community Council of Greater New York and the New York City Department of Social Services, with the aid of a grant from the Children's Bureau, United States Department of Health, Education, and Welfare.

The *Paths to Child Placement* study was an effort to collate systematically information about families during the year *prior* to foster care, on the assumption that this would be a useful base for planning and developing services that might prevent the need for foster care.

The primary method was extensive direct interviewing with the parents (this included employment of skilled interviewers able to communicate with parents who did not speak English). The case selection process was designed to identify for interview all families involved in a first social-agency child-placement experience between May 1 and August 31, 1963. During that period, Bureau of Child Welfare intake records indicated that roughly 2,000 children from 1,000 families came into care. Of that total, 1,069 children from 512 families met the definition for inclusion in the study.

But I am not here to tell you about how the study was done nor of details of its findings. I want rather to tell you about how the findings are being used as a springboard for getting long-overdue action toward building a more effective system of child protection in New York City—in other words, to tell you that study recommendations have led to results! How significant they are you will have to judge for yourselves, as I tell you briefly about them. Even a small success in effecting a change in child protection practice seems unusual enough—in New York City—to make it worthwhile for me to tell you a little about what we are doing, how we got started, and where we hope to go from here.

Perhaps it was the remembrance of good studies gathering dust that strengthened the Community Council's determination that with this study it would be different. Perhaps the action-promise was built into the study design itself in its methodology, which included a garnering of parents' own words. The lay Chairman of the Study Advisory Committee suggests this. In her letter of presentation at the beginning of the study report, Mrs. Richard J. Bernhard concludes with these sentences:

> The Report tells what these parents have said about their life situations in the year prior to the first foster care experience. It is up to all of us to listen.

It was the words of the parents incorporated in the study that influenced me most as I read and re-read the study, and then decided to accept a job with the Community Council as study "implementer." Over and over, they described child-rearing efforts against the terrible odds of poverty, severely deteriorated housing, annual pregnancies, discrimination, and absence of a strong family to fall back on, in many instances, of even a spouse. Parental illness—physical and mental—was the major problem leading to child placement for more than half the families, and a contributing factor in many of the others. Name the social pathology—whether it be desertion, illegitimacy, drug addiction, alcoholism, poverty, or child neglect or abuse—and you will find it in abundance in the population of families whose children come into care in New York City on a crisis basis. And the crisis route, the study showed, is the way the majority of children *do* come into foster care.

The study recommendations to be implemented covered the waterfront of action needed in mental health, in the schools, and in all aspects of social welfare service. There was also a call for better case planning and coordination between and within agencies. The study, indeed, in addition to pinpointing circumstances that lead to parental failure, also provided insights into obvious shortcomings or failure in the community "system" for assuring help to families and timely protection for children.

Most alarming to me, as I read and re-read the case stories and studied the data, was the clear evidence that many of the children were in desperate need for community protection and concern for a year—and often much longer than that—before the community machinery for providing foster care finally ground into action. I kept coming back to one thought. The study focus on the placement issue, and therefore, the major action goal—prevention of placement—was too narrow. The case situations reported seemed to me to cry for action toward the much broader goal of building a comprehensive network of child-care and protection services and of assuring their availability on the scale and in the places needed.

Placement for some children could certainly have been avoided. For others of the children described, placement was clearly needed the day they were born, and planning for it should have been completed even before that. Some mothers reported having found "alternatives to placement" that appeared to me to be indescribably unsuitable and too hazardous for the community to ignore or tolerate. The fact that large numbers of the children were back home within three months decreased the "in-placement" totals, to be sure, and was a good thing for some, but a bad thing for others. Missing in most of the descriptions was evidence of a viable community concern, expressed in a realistic "system" for assuring social protection to *all* children in jeopardy and help to parents, at the time and of the kind that was needed.

All in all, the study findings and the thinking I did about them helped clarify and fill out for me a picture of a community unprepared and ill-equipped to deal in a basic and comprehensive way with its massive problems of child protection. Even planning and service around the issue of placement appeared timed to begin *after* a child is already out of his home, instead of before. A wide range of services and resources seemed clearly needed, and not available in anything like the quantity or at the time or in the places required. Moreover, the many related service "systems" affecting the well-being of children appeared to be operating independently of each other, with no evidence of an overall plan for effective coordination. For example, a walk-in psychiatric clinic that recognized a mother's need for help arranged for her hospitalization on an emergency basis. A few nights later, neighbors called the police to report that the alcoholic neighbor in whose care the distraught mother had left the children had not been home for two days. The police found three children alone, hungry, and terrified, in a dark, rat-and roach-infested apartment. Since the community emergency shelter care "system" divided up families of children in accordance with their age or sex, the police took one child to the New York Foundling Hospital, one to the Bureau of Child Welfare's Children's Center, and the other to the third major public shelter facility, Callagy Hall.

Or, for another example, in family after family, it was that most predictable of emergencies, confinement, that seemed to come regularly and as a great surprise, and that precipitated this same kind of nighttime emergency procedure. It was clear in many cases that the mother's approaching need for hospitalization and for child care help was known long in advance, and should have been obvious, to several community agencies.

Bringing about action to remedy all the ills in the child care and protection system began to seem, more and more, to be a gigantic project. Obviously, I thought, it is not a one-person, nor a two-year job. I won't recount all the steps in the process of assembling a powerful committee of lay and professional persons and getting ready for the first meeting with the Committee. Essentially, I tried to recast the Study findings into encompassable problem terms. Three problems stood out as targets against which action needed to be directed:

Problem I

> Entry to foster care, more often than would be necessary, comes about on a crisis basis, which is costly to the community and dangerous to children.

Problem II

> Children caught in unavoidable crises are suffering greater damage than is necessary or than is economical. Crisis situations cannot always be anticipated, prepared for, or avoided. They can be "cushioned," however, and their potential for damage can be diluted.

Problem III

> Children are coming into care much too late, often after family deterioration is far advanced and after serious and possibly irreversible child damage has already occurred.

After each one of these problems was a detailed description of the specific program "actions" that I believed were required. This was further spelled out in a listing of the specific services that would have to be developed or further expanded in order to do this. I prepared a chart listing and describing what I saw as the essential social services a community should provide.

The major purpose of the chart and proposals was to spell out and try to get agreement on the totality of the job to be done. It was also important to divide the totality into its many parts. This was essential in order for the Committee to consider where to start, or what part to take hold of first.

Perhaps my spate of written words sent in advance of the meeting served a good purpose. At the time of the first Committee meeting, Committee members all felt the same need to say everything on their minds—related or not related to the study, to the written plan proposals, or to the agenda. The final words said, however, were loud and clear and right on target. The Committee wanted to start! They wanted to cause *something* to happen. They were afraid this Committee, like others, would get bogged down in mere talk about the totality of the problem and the size of the challenge. If it was a commitment to all-out development of a comprehensive network of services that we needed, fine; they were committed, and so voted without a dissent. They wanted, however, to start at once toward this large goal, by doing something to change the picture of the large numbers of children experiencing placement for the first time on an emergency basis, in the middle of the night, with police, not social workers, initiating the idea and bringing them in police cars to large congregate shelters. (The fact that the congregate shelter care "system" separated family groups according to age and sex, added to the bleak nighttime picture.)

> "If nothing else is done," a spokesman for this choice said, "let's at least get a nighttime telephone number to the Social Services Department, so that the police have a number to call to contact the persons who will be responsible for case work planning, so that at least the planning can start *before* the child is removed from his home, instead of afterwards, and by daylight instead of in the middle of the night."

As you must know, nothing is ever so simple or so rational as that in our business. Connecting a telephone is one thing, but making needed provisions for a suitable someone to answer it and assuring that that someone will have something to offer when he does answer is something else again.

But let me tell you what has actually happened—what change has taken place—since that first Committee meeting on October 13, 1966, or what results we can actually report as of today. For one thing—and it is no small thing—the City Department of Social Services decided to have 700 homemakers on its payroll instead of 350!

But most exciting is the nighttime and weekend emergency child welfare service, which the Department put into action at 5:00 P.M. on Monday, May 22, 1967 and has kept functioning without pause since that night. The police, the hospitals, and others faced with after-hours' emergencies involving children now have a Child Welfare Services Agency to call. It is centrally located in Manhattan but responds to child care and protection emergencies throughout the five boroughs, and on a 24-hour basis. A telephone call to the After-Hours' Emergency Child Welfare Services reaches an office at the Department of Social Services. A mature social worker, who qualifies as a supervisor in the child welfare program, is on duty. After assessing the situation as well as is possible by telephone, one of these professional workers dispatches an emergency "night-watcher," or "child-sitter," to stay with the children for the remainder of the night, and to do whatever can be done to comfort the children and "cushion" the crisis for them until the next morning, when alternative parental care possibilities may be calmly considered.

The intent of the after-hours service is to "cushion" family crisis situations for children in every way possible and also to introduce casework help and thoughtful planning into the situation *before* a decision is made that a child must leave his own home. Whenever it is possible to sustain a child in his own home, this is the first choice, particularly for the large numbers of children whose need for care arises from parental illness or temporary hospitalization.

An analysis of families and children reached by the after-hours and weekend service during its first 77 days startled the Committee and the Department. The service responded to 350 family situations, involving 729 children. A precipitous middle-of-the-night placement was averted for 449 of those children, or 62%. Numbers served more than doubled, we were told, during the second two months of operation. The impact of the program on the crowded shelters is dramatically reflected in a comparison of population figures for October 15, 1966 and for October 15, 1967, a year later.

Children in custodial care

	October 15, 1966	October 15, 1967	Capacity
Children's Center	406	308	323
Callagy Hall	129	108	128
Callagy Annex	64	53	70

Exactly comparable figures are not at my fingertips for the New York Foundling Hospital but the Committee representative from that agency has reported a conspicuous and comparable drop in population figures there.

The introduction of more thoughtful assessment and planning at the point of crisis, as might be expected, has dramatized the need for greatly strengthened family counseling, as well as psychiatric services, and a range of other supportive services and resources for caseworkers to draw upon, on the "morning after." As mentioned, a beginning has been made with expanded homemaker services. Much more needs to be done in this area. More day care expansion is another obvious need.

The Department is also developing neighborhood-based foster family homes for emergency and short-time shelter care, to be used when indicated as an alternative to placement in a large congregate care institution. Advantages for the child in remaining in his own familiar neighborhood, near his school, etc., are obvious. Perhaps most important for planning purposes is the improved image potential it offers to the Department of Social Services at the neighborhood level. A realistic program of protection for all children in jeopardy—or any parent in need of help—requires that the public child welfare authority be a well-known and respected "helping" service, with high visibility and easy accessibility at the neighborhood level.

As progress is made in developing crisis-oriented services and resources, it should seem obvious to planners that it makes even better sense to make these crisis services and resources available as needed *before* a crisis occurs!

Many of our proposals, and for that reason most of our "action" thus far, has been directed toward expansion of services under public agency auspices. This is where the basic essential social services are least developed in New York City, and where they must be developed on a vastly accelerated scale in New York City—as elsewhere—if we are to achieve the goal of comprehensive coverage in relation to total need. This cannot be done in New York City without the whole-hearted support, understanding, and enthusiasm of voluntary as well as public agency leadership. The combined resources and unified planning of all are desperately needed. This, of course, includes planning with mental health agencies, with schools, and with the many other "parts" and related "pieces" of our fractionated "machinery" for helping children to grow up safe and strong.

It is too early to really evaluate either the methods or the results in this project to implement the findings and recommendations of the *Paths to Child Placement* study. The methodology is not fixed or frozen, and it is under continuous critical scrutiny. I am convinced at this point, however, that we have identified some of the most important basic ingredients for any effective "action" effort. First and foremost must be a social policy conviction that can be effectively communicated in philosophic as well as program and service terms. There must be backing from powerful professional as well as citizens' groups. It helps to have a written plan, and a timetable that envisions the totality of the task, the separate parts, and also the relationship of each to the other.

Although this project is carried on with the conviction that the project, itself, can and will make a difference, real results in New York City will reflect the efforts of many persons and organizations going on concurrently as well as over a longer period of time. No effort is being wasted, therefore, over concern for who does or does not get the credit.